the **JOYFUL CAREGIVER**

ADVANCE PRAISE

The Joyful Caregiver is a must read for anyone who is caring for a loved one. Josephine Grace has written a practical guide to help the caregiver cope with the changes that this role can bring to your life. As a home care agency owner and an oncology physical therapist I know caring for someone with a chronic or terminal illness is hard! I have seen so many people under extreme stress and burn out, with the burden of the day to day work of caring for their loved one. This book validates those feelings and emphasizes the importance of self-care and support. Ms. Grace offers ways to manage stress and taking care of yourself to allow you to effectively care for your loved one. I love that she includes the importance of finding life outside of your caregiving role so that as a caregiver the joy of life is not forgotten. If you are caring for a loved one, I strongly suggest you read this book."

– Shelia Whiteman DPT
Doctor of Physical Therapy

"Josephine Grace's book *The Joyful Caregiver* provides caregivers a comprehensive, thoughtful and loving protocol for how to manage the challenge of caring for loved ones while avoiding personal burnout. Ms. Grace offers first-hand knowledge based on her own experience of caregiving for her parents from the time she was a young girl. The wisdom and insight offered in her pages are a balm for the caregiver soul! As a psychotherapist, I would recommend this book without question, because it lets caregivers know: "You are not alone.""

– Amy Carpenter
Licensed Clinical Social Worker

"The Joyful Caregiver provides a path toward healing and understanding for those living with a loved one who has a chronic illness. Josephine has provided a wealth of resources and teaches the value of self-love using easy and practical steps. I highly recommend this exceptional guide to everyone."

– Darlene Burridge
Family Caregiver

"If you feel overwhelmed and alone and want to know how to better handle caring for your loved one, this guide will help you immensely. Josephine offers powerful, practical and solid advice on ways to be the best caregiver with confidence. This valuable resource should be available at all hospitals for caregivers. Highly Recommended!!"

– Lina Betancur
Best-selling Author

"Wish I had been able to have had this guide in the days when I had this role. I highly recommend this be a "go to" book for everyone to read. I also recommend you don't wait until you are in the thick of a situation to read this book. If you are connected with any kind of caregiving support group, this should be your number one gift for everyone. I highly recommend it."

– Jennifer Brooks
Former Caregiver

"This is a beautiful and empowering book for those faced with caring for a loved one. It gives the caregiver the resources and knowledge to care for themselves while caring for others. The steps provided to better yourself are extremely valuable. Teaching you to be positive and constructive while your loved ones are recovering and filling up with gratitude during and after their care. It offers many resources and tools for personal growth. Thank you to Josephine Grace for sharing her life experiences as a caregiver and for giving hope to those who are now caregivers. I really wish I had this book 17 years ago, so that I could share with my mother the steps that may have made her life as a primary caregiver to my father a little less stressful. Watching your loved ones suffer with a disease is difficult, but seeing the person who is caring for them lose themselves along the way, is just as hard."

– Lucy F. Nobrega
Father diagnosed with cancer

JOSEPHINE GRACE

the JOYFUL CAREGIVER

8
STEPS TO PREVENT CAREGIVER BURNOUT

NEW YORK

LONDON • NASHVILLE • MELBOURNE • VANCOUVER

The Joyful Caregiver

8 Steps to Prevent Caregiver Burnout

© 2021 Josephine Grace Petrolo

Published in New York, New York, by Morgan James Publishing in partnership with Difference Press. Morgan James is a trademark of Morgan James, LLC.
www.MorganJamesPublishing.com

ISBN 9781631950513 paperback
ISBN 9781631950520 eBook
ISBN 9781631950537 audiobook
Library of Congress Control Number: 2020936691

Cover Design Concept:	**Editor:**
Nakita Duncan	Emily Tuttle
Cover Design by:	**Book Coaching:**
Megan Dillon	The Author Incubator
megan@creativeninjadesigns.com	
Interior Design by:	**Author Photo by:**
Christopher Kirk	Josephine Grace Petrolo
www.GFSstudio.com	

DISCLAIMER

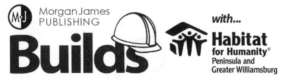

Morgan James is a proud partner of Habitat for Humanity Peninsula and Greater Williamsburg. Partners in building since 2006.

Get involved today! Visit
MorganJamesPublishing.com/giving-back

To Mom, thank you for believing in miracles
and for never giving up on me.
You are my Sunshine!

Mom and Dad, thank you for teaching me compassion,
devotion and resilience. I am eternally grateful.

Patty, thank you for being the inspiration to write this book.
I hope you're dancing with joy!

And to all the caregivers in the world, may you discover a new
level of awareness and self-love through reading this book.

In gratitude and reverence,
I love you.

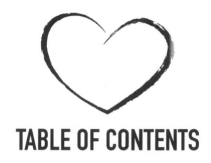

TABLE OF CONTENTS

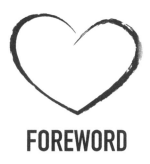

FOREWORD

As a Family Medicine Physician, I am so grateful that Josephine Grace wrote a book on helping myself and others understand the challenges that caregivers face. Before reading this book, I did not know how it felt to be that person, to deal with the emotional and situational challenges that come with caring for someone with a disease on a daily basis. *The Joyful Caregiver* helped me to know what skills to learn and prioritize when faced with what feels like an insurmountable and painful situation with no known endpoint. It offers the importance of transforming one's frame of reference while also giving the concrete tools on how to manage this important and challenging work. As it connects squarely with those who have fallen into the courageous role as caregiver, its wisdom extends equally well to those facing any difficult challenge in life.

Josephine Grace shines a light of love and hope in what will certainly be one of the darkest times in a person's life who cares for a loved one with cancer. Her deep understanding of the path caregivers face beautifully blends with her expertise as a life coach. Whether you have just found out about the diagnosis of a disease in a loved one, have become the unexpected caregiver, or are well on the road for caring for a loved one, this book will help you to find the power within you to know you can care for your loved one, while also thrive in your own life.

– Dr. Christopher Yee
Seattle, Washington

Chapter 1:

TIME IS RUNNING OUT!

Caregivers go through more than they will tell you.
They give up a lot and rarely have a social life.
They can get sick and emotionally worn out.
It's a lot for one person. We never really know
until we walk the path of a caregiver ourselves.
- Understanding Compassion

I wrote this book for you. I understand and know what you're going through. The experience of being a caregiver can be complex, confusing, and challenging, but it can also be rewarding when you are provided with resources, tools, and support.

Meet Serena, whom I've coached through her dad's battle with cancer. She writes:

> *I am thirty-five years old, single, self-employed, and mourning my mom's death. Truth be told, I don't think I have time to mourn her death. My dad was diagnosed with cancer a few years ago, and now I've become his advocate and caregiver. I need to be a pillar of strength for him. I wonder what it's like to lose your spouse after fifty years of marriage? He's become more devout to his faith, and my relationship with God has certainly deepened during these trying times. Every morning and every night, my dad and I talk, and before bed, we speak on the phone and pray together. I look forward to the calls with my dad.*
>
> *I promised Mom, right before she transitioned over to the next realm, that I would take good care of dad. This past year has been extremely challenging. I had a nervous breakdown. My ex fiancé broke off our engagement (over the phone, I might add!). I was laid off work (wrongful dismissal according to my lawyer, but I was too distraught to fight it). My mom had been in and out of hospitals (I was by her bedside most of the time when I wasn't at work), and my dad's health deteriorated. But I had to keep it together for them. Being a caregiver for your parents isn't easy, and I've burned my candle at both ends many times.*

Years ago, I took a trip to Costa Rica for four months to recharge. It's difficult now to take any trips because my dad depends on me. He's in a fragile state, and I made a promise to my mom that I would be by his side and take good care of him. I don't exactly agree with the radiation cancer treatment. I've been down this road before with Mom and her prescriptions protocol. How can radiation and prescription drugs build your immune system? There's no way! They suppress the symptoms; they don't do anything with dealing with the root cause! It actually does the opposite. These doctors aren't even open to the alternatives! They look at me like I'm from Mars when I even bring up any alternative medicine approaches. "Dad, there are other alternatives to cure you from cancer." I've had these conversations often. He just wants to heal from his pain and discomfort at this point. He made the decision to go with the radiation and surgery route, and although I don't agree, I need to stay strong and support him. I've forgotten what it's like to have fun. I keep thinking about my mom. I knew she was going to pass away that night and yet I chose to leave the hospital because I was exhausted. Thankfully, I convinced my brother to stay by mom's bedside. I wasn't surprised when I received the phone call at 5:00 am the next morning.

I spend most of my time in survival mode, trying to find ways to pay my bills and be the best caregiver for my dad. That's the beauty of being an entrepreneur. I set my own time and schedule because I need to be flexible for all the doctors' appointments and time spent with dad. My social life is on hold. I don't have a television, and most of my spare time I read inspirational self-help books, entrepreneur business startup books, or anything to do with self-improvement and having a healthy lifestyle. I love going for long walks with my dog, spending time in nature, and reflecting on life. Talking with God often has become a priority. He always has my back, and I'm grateful for that. How am I going to stay strong for my dad? I don't want to have another breakdown. How can I be the best caregiver for him? How do I support his decision for conventional methods when there's a whole world out there that he hasn't tapped into? All these questions run through my head all the time! I barely sleep.

Serena came to me distraught and asking for help. She wanted to know how to better handle taking care of her dad so she could help him beat cancer. I started this journey with her, met her where she was, and helped her create a road map with tools and resources to help her dad get the care and support he needed to defeat cancer. In the process, she reconnected with herself and spirit, became self-compassionate, and experienced acceptance and healing. Her levels of anxiety and panic attacks went away, and her dad received the support he needed to navigate his journey.

Maybe your story sounds like Serena's. Maybe you're a caregiver for a loved one who is chronically sick or has a chronic disease. The wisdom in this book can be applied to all caregivers and their loved ones. The action steps Serena took to better handle taking care of her dad are the same steps that can be applied in your life to better care for yourself and your loved one. These are wellness principles and skills that you will use for the rest of your life.

Today, Serena is doing well. She's a vibrant entrepreneur and wellness advocate living her best life and helping others do the same. She started her journey on her own until she realized she could ask for support. This can be you: implementing new ways to handle your loved one's care so that they receive the help they need to defeat the disease and you live your best life possible during your caregiving journey.

Chapter 2:

HOW DO I TAKE BETTER CARE OF MY LOVED ONE?

"The capacity to care is the thing that gives life its deepest significance and meaning."
- Pablo Casals

Nine months ago, my friend Patty died, and I didn't even know she was sick. She had cancer. I found out a week before she died that she was in palliative care at the hospital from a mutual friend. I don't know why this hit me hard, but it did. I felt the pain and suffering that my friend was going through. You see, nine years ago, my dad passed away with cancer. And what Patty and I shared is we were caregivers for our parents. There was always a bond between Patty and I. We would share conversations and discuss the challenges of being a caregiver. We always thought we were alone in this process until we realized it was one we shared. It was a difficult journey.

Patty died of cancer on her forty-fourth birthday. I didn't even know she was suffering! I would have loved to have a conversation about this with her and to be there for her when she needed it most. But, I didn't have that opportunity. I only communicate with her now through the ether. At the same time, our mutual friend Stef was in pain and suffering too. She didn't forgive Patty for something years before, and she held a grudge for so long, even when Patty reached out several times to apologize and ask for forgiveness. However, Stef was stubborn and chose not to forgive her. So when Stef called me with the news that Patty was in the hospital, she was upset and sad that she didn't have the opportunity to speak with Patty. You see, she did go to the hospital to visit Patty when she found out the severity of her illness. Patty only had limited time to live. At the door, she was stopped by Patty's mom, who basically yelled at her and told her to leave. "How dare you come to the hospital when Patty's on her death bed. Where were you all these years? You treated my daughter so poorly, even when she reached out to you. You caused her so much pain and grief, and now you're here? Leave! You are not allowed to enter her room." So, my friend left with remorse and tears down her face. To this day, she is still going through this and doesn't have peace of mind which leads me back to why I wrote this book.

Cancer or any form of chronic disease is very challenging, especially if you're advocating for a loved one. Essentially, as caregivers, you believe that their life depends on you. Living your life with that belief and burden is stressful. I'm here to share that I've been there. I understand what you're going through. You're not alone. I've gone through what you are going through now, and I want you to know that I'm here for you. This book will bring you a new level of awareness, a deeper understanding of the Power within you that is greater than any situation, condition, or circumstance. You have the opportunity to activate that Power within you and truly become a leader, advocating for you and your loved one's life. Both of you matter in this process, and in order for you to understand this, you need someone who has gone through it before you to shed some light and provide you with a roadmap of options and considerations to help guide you on your loved one's wellness journey. I'm here to love you and support you during this challenging time.

Disease is simply that—dis-ease. When you learn ways to release all dis-ease, through thoughts and lifestyle changes, you will welcome health, love, and happiness into your life. We often hear about self-love, yet we've never been exposed to it or learned ways to practice it for ourselves or others. For over twenty years, I've studied ways to better myself and to serve and help my parents, diving deep into why their dis-ease occurred in the first place and if it's really true that genetics are the main driving force for health.

I'm thrilled to know today that there are many physicians and scientists who have discovered that this is not true. Genes aren't the main driving force for health. We have the power to change our "disease reality" into "truth and wellbeing reality." This is what I would love for you to experience, and I invite you to be open, do your own research, and know that there is an Infinite Intelligence that is breathing you, the same Intelligence that will help you through this difficult time and for the rest of your life. I'm here to support you and show you ways to activate this intelligence and power within you.

I was born a caregiver, so I was told by my mom. I always thought and believed this was true, so I lived my life choosing her needs before mine at times—not always, but when I didn't, I felt guilty that I wasn't choosing her needs first. I always had this either/or mentality. Twenty years later, after I met my mentor, Mary, I realized that there is a way to create both/and scenarios, and I want to teach and show you the way. This is what I would have loved to share with Patty, yet I wasn't given the opportunity to help her. I'm given the opportunity to help you, so I'm doing this for you and for all the compassionate and devoted caregivers. This book will help reduce the stress in your life so that you can be a joyful caregiver and live your best life.

You may read some of this book and ask yourself, *Can I do this? Would this really make a difference? Can my loved one really defeat disease?* Well, let me share with you… When you agree with the prognosis and start living your life according to the prognosis, then the condition has already defeated you. In other words, the moment one hears that they have a dis-ease, they freak out, fear creeps in, and they start living or essentially dying. There isn't peace of mind, only fear that becomes the driving force to their decisions and lifestyle. Essentially, they've given up. For a very long time, many have radically underestimated our body's power to transform and restore back to health. I'm here to share never, ever, ever give up on yourself or your loved one! Our body has the power to heal and recover with the right support.

Over twenty years ago, my mother's prognosis was she had six months to live. The doctor called me into her room and told me to prepare for the inevitable because my mom was going to die. I was furious with the doctor, and I yelled, "Who in the world do you think you are, God!? Unless you're planning to kill her, you have no right to tell me she has six months to live!" And at that moment, I realized what had just come out of my mouth. I also want to share with you that from that moment forward, I was determined to up-level my research, determination, and willingness to help Mom live longer than six months. I just knew in my heart there was another way. That was the kick-start for my health and wellness journey. I read books, became a Reiki practitioner, studied nutrition, became an aromatherapist, and studied several healing modalities to help my mom through her journey, and be the best caregiver. I am grateful and appreciative to say that my mom lived for another twelve years! My caregiver journey then continued with my dad when he was diagnosed with cancer. He lived battling cancer for four years. The tools and strategies I learned to cope and navigate my mom's health helped me through the caregiving challenges with my dad. These principles shared in this book, are lifelong skills that any caregiver can apply to their life.

Another important lesson I learned was the importance of creating a safe and supportive environment for our loved ones regardless of what we think is best for them. We can provide our loved ones with resources, information, and tools. We may also learn new ways of treating their condition which they may or may not agree to do. Ultimately, it is their decision, and we need to respect their wishes. Serena's story is a great example—she did not agree with her father's decision to do radiation and surgery. This alone can cause stress both for her and her family. She had to learn ways to respect and accept her parent's wishes, regardless of what she felt was the right thing for them. No one can predict what could happen. There is a fine line between being someone's health advocate while ensuring they have the help they need and want, and providing them with the best care possible, without giving up on them.

There is a way to live gracefully and experience happiness in your life on this difficult journey navigating disease with your loved one. I'm not here to tell you it's easy or that you should be content that your loved one has a chronic condition. I'm here to share with you ways to reduce the stress and be compassionate, resilient, joyful and empowered.

If you practice these steps, you, along with those around you, will see the transformation of light, love, compassion, and improved relationships. You will find the Power within you to help you through the turbulent times. You will have tools and strategies to ensure your loved one receives the care and help they need. You will be guided to the best ways to handle your self-care and encouraged to make yourself a priority. Your health and life matters too! You can be joyful and prevent caregiver burnout.

Chapter 3:

8 STEPS—THE GRACEFUL PROCESS™

Congratulations on taking the first step toward victory! By simply choosing to read this book, you have taken a huge step toward transformation, joy and preventing burnout. You have chosen to take "time out" from your caregiving responsibilities to do something for yourself. This is often the most difficult step of all. Finding a way to make time to do this probably took a lot of effort, and you will soon begin to see the rewards for your efforts.

Every day, the aging of a loved one presents immediate caregiving challenges to spouses, children, and other family members who are suddenly forced into the role of caregiver in the midst of chaos. In many cases, your need to serve as a caregiver will just be temporary until your loved one recovers.

In other cases, however, you transition and serve as a long-term caregiver.

Short-term or long-term, all caregivers run the risk of burnout if they don't care for themselves properly first in order to be able to effectively care for others. Caregivers are heroes, looking after loved ones around the clock often with little help and few financial resources. No matter what your personal circumstances, caregiving can start to take its toll when you don't know the warning signs of caregiver burnout and how to prevent it. You miss your life. You're hurting. How do you keep your life during a life of caregiving?

Caregiver burnout is mentally, physically, and emotionally exhausting and occurs when the caregiver isn't getting the help they need. This book will show you ways to have a life with joy while caregiving. This information is here to help alleviate the stress and burdens of being a caregiver and provide you with *soul*utions to navigate your health along with your loved one's health, with grace and ease.

As a caregiver, I was so affected by my parents' disease and death. The serious illness occurs to the entire family, not just the parents. When a loved one is sick, it sends waves of emotion throughout the extended family system, changing the dynamics of relationships. It certainly impacted and changed the dynamics within my own family. Practicing compassion, understanding, and forgiveness was critical to the health and wellbeing of my family. How well caregivers deal with the loved one's illness or disability will shape the ways they function for years to come. The resentments created when relatives argue over caregiving, or abandon each other due to lack of support or communication, have powerful impacts. On the flip side, when family members caregive together, a harmonious bond is created and strengthened during this challenging time.

I've written this book to help family members—in particular, for adult children of aging parents diagnosed with a chronic illness. This isn't to say that this book is only for caregivers whose parent is diagnosed with a disease; in fact, these steps will guide you to living your best life while navigating the care of any family member who is not well. It's about doing the right thing and practicing love and loyalty in the smartest ways possible without risking creating other family problems or dissonance. It's about advocating and giving a voice to family caregivers so they realize their lives are a priority and matter too!

The Graceful Process offers eight steps that will help you work through the roadblocks holding you back from living your best life during your loved one's battle with a chronic illness. I have personally journeyed through these steps over the twenty years of caring for my parents. These are the gems that I discovered along the way, usually through the hardship that I needed to overcome. I learned the most effective ways to navigate the adversities and challenges and now I am sharing this process with you. They will help you get better at handling stress and embracing your place in this wellness journey so you and your loved ones can live a joyful and meaningful life even in the midst of chaos.

While using this book as part of your support system, you will learn:

- ♥ How to work with your loved one's doctors.
- ♥ Ways to create a schedule that works for you and your family.
- ♥ Warning signs of caregiver burnout.
- ♥ How to become compassion resilient.
- ♥ How to care for yourself and be guilt-free.
- ♥ How to have moments of joy during this difficult time.
- ♥ How to make decisions coming from love rather than fear.
- ♥ Ways to improve your relationships.

I recommend you have your calendar, a notebook, and a pen handy as you journey along this path. Ideas and inspiration will come to you, and I encourage you to write them down in a journal.

Caregiving is one of the most difficult jobs you will ever face. Thankfully, help is here. This book is written by a caregiver for caregivers with the intention that you learn the most effective strategies for taking care of yourself first. It's an honor to share my story and experience with you, and a privilege to sprinkle you with hope. There is another way to navigate this caregiving journey. You can welcome the support and stay healthy!

Chapter 4:

STEP 1—HOW DO I WORK WITH MY LOVED ONE'S DOCTORS?

t's a challenging time, but you've got this. It may not seem that you know what to do right now, and I'm here to help you. I hear you saying how frustrating it gets when you are talking with the doctors. I encourage you to prepare for your appointments with the doctors. You want to build a health team, and the only way to do that is to prepare for it. So what does that look like?

You want to empower yourself with information. Ask questions, lots of questions. In fact, your questions will determine the care your loved one receives. Always have a notebook and pen at hand and jot the information down. Track any changes and definitely keep a list of all the medications. When my mom and dad were going through this, I accompanied them to their doctors' appointments. I had a list of questions that I asked the physicians. I asked for copies of their results. I wanted to ensure that I stayed on top of things. You want to be informed and keep a record of their health care.

It would be helpful to have some understanding of the possible options and the reasoning for the physicians' particular approach. Here are examples of specific questions that you can ask your loved one's physician:

1. What can I expect with my loved one's condition—in a week, a month, three months, a year?
2. What are the options for treatment?
3. What are the advantages and disadvantages of each option?
4. What are the medication side effects?
5. What is your reasoning for your treatment recommendations?
6. What contingency plans do you have in mind if the initial treatments are ineffective?
7. What role can I play in helping my loved one?
8. What is the best way for me to communicate with you on an ongoing basis?
9. Where can I get a second medical opinion, can you refer me to another physician?

There is an abundance of information out there, and I strongly recommend you become informed and do your research. Ultimately, you want to partner with the best heath care team that share the common medical objectives for your loved ones.

Often, I noticed that my clients were not aware they could get a copy of their results and tests. I even kept copies of the requisition forms before they were handed in to the labs. You always hear that knowledge is power, but it's the action steps you take with the knowledge that empowers you. So asking for copies of everything helps when you are doing your own research for the best care. Also, when you're building your health team, they usually ask for the results or details of the medical reports. Typically, they can get these forwarded from the doctors directly, provided you sign a release form; however, that could take time. Your best bet is to provide your team with upfront notes. Even when they're likely going to want to do their own testing, they will still have a starting point with the records you've provided.

During this time, you will experience a roller coaster of emotions. This is normal. In fact, that's the good news. These emotions come up in order for you to notice them and learn ways to navigate them. You see, we're not meant to feel any one emotion all the time. We're meant to experience the emotion fully and then let it go.

Take, for example, my outburst with the doctor when he shared with me that my mom had six months to live. After those words came out, I thought, *what in the world did I just say?* My mom's life is dependent on the care of this doctor. Part of me was glad this outburst came out. I mean, it's true. How could they determine the exact timing when someone is going to die? Based on statistics? Well, I can assure you I'm glad I didn't believe and follow those statistics. My mom lived for another twelve years. And that's my point; no one knows the exact date when any of us are going to die. One thing is for sure though. We've all entered into this world, and we will all have to exit this world. You will do your best to work with the team and there will be times when what they're going to share with you will be hard to hear and accept. Chances are you may have already experienced this. It is normal to feel this way. You're not alone. In fact, you will never have to feel this way on your own. You can always pick up this book and re-read it or, better still, reach out and send me an email.

It's important during this process that you build your own health care team. Choose those who you and your loved one resonate with, who you can partner with, and who you will feel comfortable asking your questions. They should be answering your questions with hopeful and real answers. Another client, Dora, her mom showed signs of breast cancer and the specialist she was working with kept dismissing her questions and the suggestion that she wanted to explore other options instead of surgery and radiation. Her doctor wasn't open to her willingness to explore. He discouraged her from seeking alternatives. She became disengaged and walked around doom and gloom thinking that she had no other options. Then we connected at a networking event, and I encouraged her to explore finding a new doctor, one who is supportive and open to partnering with her and her wishes.

We are our highest authority, and we know what's best for us. You want to partner with a doctor who will work with you so that you receive the best care for your loved one. Often, your loved one will feel discouraged, hopeless, and worried. Continuing to visit a doctor who isn't compassionate and open to alternatives can make you both feel even worse. Instead, seek a doctor that you like, that will provide you with information, and that will encourage you to seek information so that your loved one receives the best care and support. One day, on a coaching call with Dora, she was thrilled that she found a doctor that her mom liked, and this doctor has been helpful and compassionate. They exist! So start seeking, and build your health team.

Who are the People on Your Health Team?

They can include oncologists, nurse practitioners, family physicians, pharmacists, specialists, wellness coaches, physiotherapists, naturopathic doctors, acupuncturists, nutritionists—basically anyone you choose as your health care provider, including you! You are the primary caregiver who stays on top of your loved one's treatment. That's why it's vital you choose your team carefully and work together collaboratively. Ask for second opinions, and don't be shy. It's all in the way you ask and communicate with your team. Learning ways to effectively and gracefully communicate with others is very important in all aspects of your life and especially when lives depend on it. You want to choose the team that has your back: partners who will provide you with support and answer your questions with hope, a team that's compassionate, informed, resourceful, and open to possibilities!

Also, a big part of your team is Infinite Source. You may refer to Source as God, Buddha, Universe, Infinite Intelligence, or a Higher Power, whatever resonates with you. I want to emphasize that we are all unique, energetic beings, and we receive messages and signs from God that are unique for each of us to listen and give meaning to. Tune in and listen. Your intuition will guide you.

It's known that caregiving on your own, without a proper network of support, can lead you down a difficult path of physical and emotional exhaustion. It's true you can do anything you set your mind to, but no one person can do everything. Never be embarrassed or shy about asking your healthcare provider to re-explain something that they have said. How well you understand something will affect your ability to act on that information. See yourself as a compassionate scientist with high engagement in taking care of your family member but with low attachment to the outcome. Often, caregivers are empaths. They pick up the joy, pain, and suffering that is around them. You will learn ways in the upcoming chapters on how to care for yourself in this process so that you can be your best too. Being an advocate for your loved one isn't easy; it can be complex, confusing, and challenging - but also very rewarding.

Good communication with your health team, and keeping records up to date will help you care for your loved one and keep doctors informed of any changes and results. Keep a doctor's visit journal and encourage your loved one to keep a journal of his or her own daily activities, including any symptoms. Point form is better than not having anything jotted down. It's more challenging to recall specifics by memory and much easier to have a reference point with dates and times.

Here are some support links that I've found useful. There are many out there, you can use these as a starting point:

- ♥ www.tevacaregivers.com
- ♥ www.caregiverslibrary.org
- ♥ www.agingcare.com
- ♥ www.thecaregiverspace.org
- ♥ www.caregiver.org

A diagnosis of a disease is the first step in mapping out the treatment and care for your loved one. For some, having an explanation of the symptoms brings a sense of sadness but relief. A proper diagnosis offers a chance to get help and plan for the future. Forming partnerships with doctors can also help, and you can start by understanding the disease and its treatment. Also, stay open to new possibilities. I'll elaborate more on this in future chapters.

Partnering, asking questions, and providing information to the doctors and other care providers can improve your loved one's care. Sharing information with your health team builds trust and leads to better results, quality of life, safety, and possibilities. Consider starting a closed Facebook group or a blog to keep the health care team and family informed and updated on their care. Remember, effective communication and jotting down notes will help the team offer best solutions.

Listen, doctors don't have much time to spend with their patients. It's sad and true. That's why it's important for you to be prepared, informed, and ask questions during your appointments. It will also be important to cultivate relationships with the nurses. They generally have inside scoops that will help with your loved one's care, including doctor referrals. If you're seeking a doctor for your loved one, nurses will have some really good advice on doctors. It's a starting point. Then, of course, make sure you follow-up, and you resonate with the doctor before involving too much energy with setting up appointments for your family. Remember, when you're keeping notes and copies of lab results, ask relevant questions. The health care team will see how involved you are in your loved one's care, and there's a better chance that they will become more involved too. This will keep medical errors at a low risk. Yes, we're all humans, and we all make mistakes. Let's pay attention to details and lessen that chance.

Caregiving is about being an informed, engaged, and proactive advocate. If you don't get the answer you're seeking from the team, ask the question in another way until you're satisfied. Then, you may get a response you can interpret and understand, even if it's not as direct as you would have liked.

Many doctors are reluctant to make a recommendation. They want the patient to be the decision-maker to avoid feeling responsible if the results don't turn out to be positive. Sometimes they remain neutral when they truly do not know which option is best. The doctor's role is to de-personalize and detach from what they're doing, but when you ask them a certain question, it forces them to answer you in a very personal way. Don't be afraid to ask, "What if they were your parent or a really close family member? What would you recommend?" Chances are high that you'll receive a more realistic response.

No one has to go on their journey alone. I recommend that someone always be beside your loved one when they are going to their appointments or treatments. Whether it's you, another family member, a friend, someone from work, your business partner, or hired help. Keeping a watchful eye on your loved one's medical professionals is important because when a patient is hospitalized, their care involves so many different people and not everyone has the time to read the patient's records carefully. You also need to get copies of the medical records that follow your loved one through the various stages of their care. The health care system has many medical professionals or personnel that transfers information and care from one to another. This creates plenty of opportunity for information to be lost, recorded incorrectly, or simply overlooked.

I recall a time when my mother entered a surgery room and was being prepared for surgery. One nurse (whom I call an angel) stated her name incorrectly—it was almost her exact last name but one letter off, and my mom raised her voice to pronounce her own name correctly. The nurse apologized and said my mother actually was not the correct patient for the surgery. According to my mom, everyone in the surgery room scattered, and she was returned to her hospital room. How frightening is that? Imagine you're in a hospital, and usually on your own for surgery, and you're the wrong patient in the surgery room!

Needless to say, I worked really hard at managing my emotions when I heard this! I had to treat them in a respectful manner while I was furious with what happened. Holding back without anger is a challenge when you're so emotionally engaged in helping your loved one through a difficult experience. As soon as you start yelling, people tune you out. I tried very hard to stay as calm and articulate as I could be and get my point across. If you do that enough times, people have a certain level of respect for your credibility. That way, if you do lose control of your emotions once, they won't hold it against you.

Bottom line, if you feel too emotionally engaged to sustain a good balance, consider bringing in a more objective third party to help with the care—a therapist, a friend, or relative who has some medical or mediation training. I love consulting with physician friends who look at patients as a whole person, incorporate both medical and complementary forms of treatment, and are open to partnering with me and my family instead of dictating what to do and not do. I've experienced both types of physicians, and I choose those whom I resonate with and who align with my own research and values. Having all the information presented and trusting that I will receive all the answers I need, helps me make informed decisions for myself and my loved one on our wellness journey.

Chapter 5

STEP 2—WHAT DO I DO AND WHEN?

Stop! Just breathe. Everything is going to be alright. You put so much pressure on caring for your loved one that you've created a codependent cycle of madness. You are not responsible for their life. You've placed so much pressure on yourself! Stop worrying and making yourself anxious. Your loved one has their own path, and you are here to be by their side and leave the rest to their journey. What you need to do now is be present, listen, and appreciate the time you have with them. Talk to them. See what they would love to do and schedule their love list in your calendar. Do activities that would lighten them up and bring them more joy and life!

Yes, you have doctors' appointments. Yes, you have your work, but you will get through this. Breathe deeply and slow down. Stop rushing through life and missing crucial points of inner wisdom because you're moving too fast to listen and tune in. There's a gift in everything! When it looks like bad things are happening, in reality, things are simply happening, and you give them meaning. You call them bad or good. Therefore, focus on finding the good in everything happening around you.

I invite you to give this a chance and see your life change in great ways. I know that right now it's hard to see the light. You see the darkness based on what you've heard about the disease. There is hope and light even in such a debilitating disease as cancer. You see, we all have cancer cells in us. Many people don't realize this. Cancer cells grow within our body through our lifestyle, thoughts, feelings, and habits. That's a whole other picture and, quite frankly, a reprogramming conversation!

Let's stay connected with the question at hand: what do I do and when? Well, the best way to start is by creating a schedule for you and your parent. Both of you need a routine and structured schedule in order to know how you will navigate all your appointments, errands, work, etc. I encourage you to also schedule in blocks of time for fun, rest, self-care, and exercise. These should be non-negotiable and will help you stay strong and supportive, especially when you're faced with challenges that you need to overcome. You will need your high vibration energy to go out into the world. If you're running low on reserves, you'll have nothing left to give, so rest, recharging and rejuvenation are vital for both your own health and your loved one's health. They need you to be your very best, and if you follow the steps above, it will have a ripple effect on those around you. You will lead by example and inspire them to make decisions that are best for them and their health. That's the beauty in all of this. You will be guided to the right people, places, and things that will support you both on this journey. You're never alone, and asking for help is a strength, not a weakness.

So make a list of all the things you find fun, and better still, ask your loved one what they find fun too. That way, you can spend some fun time together and appreciate each other even more. Going to doctors' appointments and working all the time will not provide you with the energy you both need to keep going. Enjoy a wonderful dinner together, drink a cup of tea, take walks and hikes. Do things out of the ordinary that make you feel good, because when you're feeling good, you're actually fuelling your love tank and your heart with joy. After all, isn't that what we strive for? Bringing more joy, peace, and fun in our lives? We may not even realize it's possible at times. I've been there before and I'm here to tell you, it's absolutely possible!

I remember returning to university after my parents died. I attended school full-time and completed a dual-degree program. I went back in my late thirties after many years of being out of school, and I always kept this quote by Audrey Hepburn beside me, "Nothing is impossible. The word itself says, 'I'm possible.'" I love it because it reminds me to never give up. I never gave up on my mom even when her prognosis was six months. I never gave up on my studies, even when I had absolutely nothing left in me to keep moving forward, or at least, that's what I thought!

You see, our thoughts create our feelings, and I had some serious negative thinking that was programmed into my subconscious mind! My goodness, I'm glad I didn't listen and take its advice! You have no idea how many times I heard, "Give up already; it will never happen; why bother trying; you're just wasting your time!" It's all a lie. It's definitely worth it to keep moving forward. I encourage you to trust yourself to know what to do next and then do it! Your loved one will likely appreciate your organized schedule and the commitments you make with them—I know my Mom and Dad did! Eventually, they will anticipate your time together, and this will help them realize they're not alone in this process. Instead, they're with someone who is supportive and believes in them. This fosters hope.

So, let's get started. Take out your calendar now. Have a look at your non-negotiables, your fixed blocks of time that you'll likely not reschedule. For example, your sleeping time. Plan to get to bed every night at the same time and wake up at the same time every day. This will help with your body's cycle. I'll share more about this in a later chapter. Next, your loved one's doctors' appointments—will you be going to all of them? If so, you may want to schedule them sooner rather than later. Do you have any siblings who will help with your loved one's care? Or maybe you have a friend or other family members who would be willing to go with them? Again, reach out to your support team so that you can provide the best care. There will be times that you will need to be elsewhere and can't make their appointments. Be sure to ask for help in advance as soon as you know about the appointments so that others can schedule them in their calendar and lower the chance of any conflicts coming up. Again, be sure you choose someone who shares the same goals and offers hope and inspiration to your loved one. No one wants to be around anyone who has a negative attitude and hopeless approach!

Scheduling time for yourself is also critical. Scheduling blocks of time works best, but if you don't have chunks of time available due to other commitments, do the best you can and try to schedule at least an hour to do something for yourself every day. What sorts of things light you up and bring you life? What can you schedule in your calendar right now that will bring joy into your life?

The main point of this chapter is to allow you to gain insight on the value of preparing your schedule. I set aside time every Sunday to organize and plan for the upcoming week. That way I'm ready to start a brand-new week with a purpose. The goals and intentions we set for ourselves help determine the lifestyle and habits we schedule in our lives. You can either live your life by design or live your life by default! You have a choice. Choose well.

Many people live their lives waiting to die, especially when they receive a diagnosis. Immediately, they start living as if they are dying. Strange, right? Instead of waiting to die, why not live in the now and allow life to unfold as you design it? Choosing to accept and respond, instead of react. You can either decide that life is happening with you, or life is happening to you. The latter is created with a victim mentality, blaming everyone and everything for your misfortune. The former holds on to the idea that no matter what's going on in your life, what's inside of you is greater than any obstacle, disappointment or difficulty you might be facing.

I want to add that one of the most important things to do when you're asking yourself what to do and when, is to *stop*, breathe, and tune in. The answers will come to you when you lean in and expect the answers to show up. I know what you're thinking right now. *How's that possible? What do you mean they'll show up?* Ideas, promptings, and messages will show up in one form or another. You'll notice this to be true when you start paying attention and begin expecting answers once you've asked the questions. All the answers are already inside of you. Stop doubting yourself or worrying about outcomes. Stop creating worst case scenarios in your head. This will cause anxiety in you, and you'll transfer your worries and anxiety to others around you. There is no positive outcome with negative thoughts and feelings. You'll simply make yourself sick, and what good is that? Let me help you answer that… no good!

Chapter 6:

STEP 3—WHY DO I FEEL SO AWFUL?

"Compassion Fatigue is a state experienced by those helping people or animals in distress; it is an extreme state of tension and preoccupation with the suffering of those being helped to the degree that it can create a secondary traumatic stress for the helper."
– Dr. Charles Figley

I had no idea there was something called compassion fatigue, yet when I heard about the symptoms, a lightbulb went off. I was so exhausted and had brain fog all the time. I didn't know what exactly was going on with me. I just knew I didn't feel like me anymore. I didn't know that these feelings were because I had compassion fatigue. This isn't a diagnosis. These are signs, and signs are good news. They help us pause, redirect, and change. They give us a second chance to live. Thank God for signs! I was losing myself while I was caring for others. Giving was no longer living.

Does This Sound Familiar?

You're tired. All you think about is taking care of your loved one. The events that happened keep happening in your head. You dream about it, you take it home with you, you're no longer fun to be around, and others may start avoiding you. You've lost your sense of self. You've run on empty and have no idea how to fill your tank! Caregiving is a huge responsibility on your shoulders, and you need a break, but you have no time to take one. You have to work and pay your bills. This is when helping others hurts. You don't feel well-equipped to do it because you're fatigued and suffer from brain fog. You think that self-care is simply a word in the dictionary.

For a friend of mine Regina, who was a caregiver for her dad, her definition of self-care was crying on her way to and from the hospital. In her own words, she had to keep herself in check because when she was at the hospital she had to show everyone that she was capable to take care of her dad. "I had to show everyone around me that I was strong and able to do the job tasks. My dad gave me the executor and personal care positions, and I was always there to meet the doctors and deal with a lot of stuff, and if I was a mess, they would have looked at me and said, do you want to talk later? I had to be present for my dad right then and there." Self-care is more than being strong for others. It involves being strong for yourself. Regina recognized that she would have "burnt out" if she didn't focus on her own health and take the opportunity for compassionate care leave from work to care for her dad.

It's extremely important to have a life outside of helping your loved one. In fact, it's critical for your health and well-being. Here are some ideas of things to do to prevent compassion fatigue:

- Go get coffee with your friends
- Watch a movie
- Go to a live theatre production
- Exercise
- Do things that keep up your sense of humour
- Fuel your body and eat life-giving foods
- Schedule an afternoon at the spa
- Go dancing
- Write a love letter
- Laugh at a comedy
- Create a new memory with your loved one

Transform fatigue before it becomes burnout!

These symptoms were uncomfortably familiar to me. I was feeling irritated and frustrated most of the time, as well as worthless and terribly sad. I was isolating myself and disconnecting from everyone around me, including my family, and nothing made sense anymore. I was suffering in silence. Everyone else's needs came first. Their survival was more important than mine. We couldn't afford to put my parents in a nursing home, and we had limited in-home care that wasn't enough for the demands of my mom's illness. We had to sell our family home to afford the nursing home expenses. I remember others thinking I was just depressed, but I had compassion fatigue. I enjoyed things in life like taking strolls, reading books under a tree, being by the ocean, admiring nature, except I was too exhausted and busy to do any of those things. I was focused on my mom and dad. So, I knew I wasn't depressed; I was fatigued. I didn't even know or think that self-care was an option. I was getting up in the morning, brushing my teeth, eating on the run—or, sometimes not eating at all and thinking that was just fine, that I could drink coffee and everything would be okay. I didn't know what self-care meant. I've learned it over the years, thankfully, and know now the connection between mind, body, and spirit.

As mentioned earlier, this pattern of caregiving began in my early childhood. I learned that it was more important to take care of others before taking care of myself. When I tried to take care of myself, I had feelings of shame, self-centredness, and selfishness. I needed to overcome this, but I didn't have the tools or understanding on my own. I didn't fill myself up, so I had a nervous breakdown. If we don't fill ourselves up, if we don't care for ourselves, we have nothing left to give.

My personal boundaries were way off. In fact, I didn't have any that I was aware of. I didn't know I could say "no" and still be liked. You see, I was also a people pleaser, pleasing everyone else except myself. I let everyone and everything into my life. Oftentimes, it was hurtful and didn't help me at all. I had this impulse to rescue anyone in need. It was a pattern that I had created on a subconscious level, unbeknownst to me! It was an internal program that provided me with fight or flight reactions, protecting me from harm. I was always in survival mode, going into reserves simply to function on a day-to-day basis. It's a rough road, believe me; I've been there. It was isolating. I had emotional outbursts, suffered from physical pain, and blamed everyone and everything else for my mood. I became addicted to looking for love in all the wrong places and was seeking validation from others. I had this veil of sadness everywhere I went because I wasn't living my full quality of life. I had constant flashbacks, reliving negative events that happened in my life, sometimes even creating negative future events that never happened! I was constantly torturing myself with these thoughts, and at that time, I didn't realize I had the power to change them.

I wasn't aware that the body, mind, and spirit were integrated. I had heard of this concept before, but what exactly did it mean? We are energetic, spiritual beings having human experiences. We have the power within us to change our thoughts, feelings, and habits. I asked myself this simple question: *Where do I start making my life better? I want to live a joyful and healthy life.*

I asked for help, and my coach suggested I create a self-care plan. Now, I know what you're thinking. I thought it too—*I don't have time.* Well, here's the truth! You have the exact same amount of time as everyone else in this world—twenty-four hours a day and seven days a week. You need to schedule time! Get up half-an-hour earlier to meditate, do yoga, go for a walk, exercise; schedule that time for yourself. It's absolutely important! As a caregiver, if you are not physically and emotionally well, you will not be able to take good care of your loved one.

Spend time with yourself to find your true north and be that authentic person you are meant to be. You will recharge and fill your tank, and as a result, you will have more energy to give to others. Your healthcare plan needs to be sustainable. This isn't a one-time "fix it" prescription; this is a lifestyle change. You are a caregiver; life keeps happening and moving forward. You have been chosen and called to have a servant's heart, and when your loved one transitions over, you will be called to another caregiving position. That's what happens. We take care of each other; that's what we're about! It's best to make yourself a priority and create the self-care plan that works best for you to fuel up and pour out to others. You will have to consciously make the time and set self-care goals. Here is a checklist and starting point to create a self-care plan:

Physical

- ♥ I eat a well-balanced diet that includes a variety of fruits and vegetables, proteins, whole grains, and healthy fats.
- ♥ I drink at least eight 8-oz. glasses of water or fluid a day (an 8x8 goal).
- ♥ I sleep well each night and wake up feeling rested.
- ♥ I exercise for thirty minutes at least three times a week.

♥ I do not smoke or use tobacco.

♥ I keep up with my own medical needs, such as getting an annual checkup from my physician, I get regular dental cleanings, and monthly massages.

What are some ways you can improve your physical well-being?

Mental and Emotional

It's important to take time for yourself each day and to keep up with activities that you enjoy. Which activities do you enjoy? Schedule in your calendar all the activities that light you up. Pick one or two of your favorite activities and make them a priority in your day-to-day life.

Listening to soothing music, dancing, playing an instrument, or singing

Reading or listening to audiobooks and podcasts

Exercising or participating in group movement classes

♥ Playing sports or board games with friends

Hiking, fishing, or other outdoor sports

Meditating or practicing yoga

Painting, drawing, or other artistic pursuits

Journaling or creative writing

Attending community events or spiritual services

Doing fun activities with friends or family

Practicing personal care, such as taking long baths, having manicures or using face masks

Cooking or baking

Watching movies or TV shows

- ♥ Playing video or computer games
- ♥ Doing yard work or gardening
- ♥ Planting a garden
- ♥ Feeding the birds
- ♥ Soaking in a bathtub infused with essential oils and Epsom salts
- ♥ Enjoying a twenty to thirty minute nap

Stay Calm Strategy

When caring for a loved one, there will be times that are difficult and emotional. It's unavoidable. Prepare for these moments by having a strategy in place to help yourself calm down if you feel anxious or overwhelmed. Having a plan in place in advance will help you better manage unexpected intense emotions.

Try the following strategies:

- ♥ Do a breathing exercise.
- ♥ Repeat a meaningful mantra, affirmation, or prayer. One of my favorite when I'm experiencing shortness of breath: "I'm okay. I can breathe. I can breathe into my next moment." This tells your nervous system that you are okay and relaxes your mind and body.
- ♥ Close your eyes and sit in silence.
- ♥ Stand up and stretch.
- ♥ Take a quick walk outside.
- ♥ Call a close friend or family member.
- ♥ Complete the following: When I feel overwhelmed I will… (respond with a stay calm strategy).

Ripple Effects

Caregiver clients often have similar responses to this question: What is the most important thing in your life? Parents, kids, spouse, work, health, love. Very rarely do they say, "I am the most important thing in my life." Yet, this is true. If you can't take care of your own happiness and wellbeing first or you can't love yourself first, how on earth are you going to take care of anyone else? How can you possibly give love to anyone else? If you can't live in gratitude and joy, how can you bring fulfillment and joy to anyone else?

Stop. Be brave. Take care of yourself first. Take moments to fill your cup. Learn to say no because helping others shouldn't hurt or cause burnout. Use empathic discernment—learn what things hurt you and learn to say, "Stop, this is hurting me. Please don't say/do that. You're hurting me." It's okay to stand up for yourself. In fact, you must stand up for yourself and be your own advocate.

Spirituality is important to cultivate and nurture, whatever that looks like for you. It's different for everyone, but the outcome is the same—peace of mind, wonder, calm, relaxation, connecting to something greater than yourself. I like to call this meditation, communicating with God, making time for introspection and prayer, and listening to the silence for answers. I see God in everything and in everyone, recognizing there is more to life than what we can physically see with our eyes.

Life is meant to be lived in joy and vibrant health. Seek ways to discover what lights you up and brings you peace of mind, joy, and love. The more vibrant we are, the brighter we shine. The brighter we shine; the more light is blasted into the world… a ripple effect of greatness!

Why Do I Feel So Awful?

You're not taking care of yourself. It takes a toll on you, mentally, physically, and spiritually. You need to have a heart of gold and mind of steel as you go through this process. I understand this well. Everyone and everything else is a priority. There is this sense of obligation and guilt if you do things for yourself, so you don't. You would rather aim to make others happy (as a people pleaser) than to include happiness for yourself. You've placed so much emphasis on providing the best care for your loved one on your own because no one else can care for them the way you can. At least, that's what you believe. Only part of this belief is accurate: you do care for your loved one. That's obvious, but I say, it's okay to ask for help and include others in the care. You'll be surprised what good can come out of this.

One of my clients, Lisa, spent at least nine hours a day helping her mom with daily tasks from bathing, to ensuring her pills were in order, to driving her mom to the doctors' appointments, to cooking for her and paying her bills. She quit her job to stay home with her mom. She believed she had to provide care and be her mom's advocate all on her own. She completely gave up her life to care for her mom. Considering outside help didn't cross her mind until she met me. Our weekly discussions had provided her with a new level of awareness. I provided her with some resources, tools, and materials from this book, and she started to implement them and take action, asking for help and allowing others in to help care for her mother. A whole new world opened up for her, and she was able to start living her life again.

Here are the most common psychological and emotional consequences I've noted that caregivers experience when caring for others. Caregivers feel:

- ♥ Caregiving has negatively affected their relationships with others.
- ♥ They have lost control of their life.
- ♥ Stressed from trying to meet responsibilities with families and work.
- ♥ Their social life has suffered.
- ♥ Hopeless. They think that there's no way to solve some of the problems they may be experiencing or there's little they can do to change important things in life.

When you realize you don't have to do this all on your own and you have courage to ask for help, a world of possibility opens up for you and reduces the stress in your life. Be kind to yourself and realize that there's help out there waiting for you to take your next steps.

Caregiver Self-Assessment

As a reference, here are some ways to check your stress level. On a scale of one to five, with one being the least stressed and five being the most stressed, how stressed are you?

What's the cause of your stress?

- ❤ I don't have enough time.
- ❤ I don't have enough money.
- ❤ I don't sleep well at night.
- ❤ The holidays.
- ❤ My other family members.
- ❤ My loved one's needs are overwhelming.
- ❤ I'm trying to keep my job.
- ❤ I'm not confident in what I'm doing.
- ❤ I haven't had a break.
- ❤ My loved one is dying.
- ❤ My loved one's health is declining.
- ❤ I don't have enough help.
- ❤ I can't afford to hire help.
- ❤ I don't have enough time for other family members.
- ❤ I am really lonely.
- ❤ I feel lost.
- ❤ I miss my life.

By identifying what's causing your stress, you become aware of possible solutions that will reduce the stress. The first step is becoming aware of your mind, body, and spiritual health. Have you scored high on your stress test? By answering yes, you now realize the importance of getting help. There are many resources available to you and I've included some resources throughout this book.

Signs of Caregiver Burnout Assessment

Answer Never, Sometimes, Frequently, or Always:

- ❤ I can't fall asleep, or I frequently wake up.

I have a lack of energy during the day.

I eat too much or too little.

I am sick more often (flus, colds, headaches).

I feel impatient, or I am easily agitated.

I feel guilty that I am not doing enough.

I have trouble concentrating on everyday simple tasks.

I am becoming more forgetful.

I stopped doing activities I used to find enjoyable.

I am more socially isolated from my friends and family.

I feel sad or depressed.

I feel anxious or worried.

I have lost interest in doing things.

If you answered "frequently" or "always" for any of the above, then it's time to seek help from a healthcare provider or your local health and social service network because you have to take care of yourself too! Building a support network is one of the most important ways to prevent burnout. It can be helpful to do an inventory of professional and family/friend supports that can help you with care tasks (TevaCaregivers.com).

Here's another reason you feel so awful that many caregivers are embarrassed to share… You've convinced yourself that it's okay to put all your attention on your loved one because one day, it's going to be all over. Part of you is relieved because finally you won't have to run around all the time to doctors and specialists and radiation and chemotherapy and the pharmacy and so on! And then, you feel guilty because you have this thought, and you certainly don't want anyone to know that you've had these thoughts.

Your relationships are suffering. Who has time to date? Now you're starting to fear that you'll never find a lifelong partner and start your own family, or maybe you already have a family, and they never see you because you're too busy spending time caring for a parent! Like everyone else isn't a priority any longer until you "figure out" the best care for your parent.

Look, no one said this process and being a caregiver was going to be easy. Whether or not you think you were born to be a caregiver, you chose to be one, or one day you just became delegated as your loved one's health advocate, one thing is for sure: you are a light warrior with a servant's heart, and you love so much that it affects you deeply when you see your loved one in pain and suffering. There's a good chance you're an empath and healer too. As an empath, you are sensitive to the world, and you feel what others around you feel. It's even more critical that you learn ways to protect yourself from this energy and keep your heart tank full of vibrant energy! To do this, you must take care of yourself too. You are a priority! Always remember this as you continue this journey with your loved ones.

Stop doubting yourself! You are blessed to have this opportunity with your loved one. Here's something you can share with them when they become negative about their condition, or when they've lost hope. Say, "Stop waiting to die! Enjoy each day, and do things you love to do. Stop worrying about your disease, the worrying keeps you away from living your life now, today, in this moment. What would you love to do today?" And go do it with them! This mindset helped me give my mom and dad the best support and hope. We had the most meaningful moments and conversations during this time.

So there you have it, light warrior! I believe in you! Keep working and moving forward, trust yourself, and access your own wisdom. The following chapters will empower you to activate this wisdom.

Available Resources

It would be impossible to provide an up-to-date list of available resources for every area in North America or even for other countries where caregivers are found. What is provided here is a generic list of people, agencies, and organizations that can provide help. Use this list as your starting point and build a list of your own. Just be sure to share it with the next caregiver you meet. No caregiver needs more help than the one who has no support and is doing everything alone.

Hospitals, Senior Centers, Support Groups, Legal Aid Services, State Units on Aging, Volunteer Programs, Ombudsman Services, In-house Respite Care, Home Chore Services, Home Health Services, Home Delivered Meals, Housekeeping Services, Area Agencies on Aging, Veteran's Affairs Offices, Senior Citizen's Services, Adult Daycare Programs, Out-of-Home Respite Care, County Extension Services, Caregiver Resource Centers, Community Health Services, County Public Health Nurses, Economic Assistance Agencies, Social Security District Offices, Service Canada Centers, State Human Services Agencies, Illness and Disability Associations, Information and Referral Agencies, Mental Health and Counseling Agencies, Illness and Disability Treatments Centers, Social Service Agencies Affiliated with Church or Associations.

You may want to start by calling the United Way, the National Council on Aging, the American Association of Retired Persons, or the Eldercare Information and Referral Service at 1-800-677-1116. (Preventing Caregiver Burnout—James & Merlene Sherman)

Chapter 7:

STEP 4—HOW DO I BECOME COMPASSION RESILIENT?

Resiliency - what a great gift! Are we born with resiliency? No. It's a learned skill and a great characteristic to master. Resilience enables you to persist in the face of challenges while remaining compassionate with your loved one. In the face of adversities, you will experience this Power within you that surpasses all circumstances and situations; a Power, at times, where you say to yourself, *Wow, I didn't know I had that within me*. It's in those defining moments that resiliency is strengthened, and a new level of awareness rises within us.

The Compassion Resilience Toolkit defines compassion resilience as "maintaining our physical, emotional, and mental wellbeing (using energy productively) while compassionately identifying and addressing the stressors that are barriers to [our loved ones]." I love this definition because it includes mind, body, spirit and recognizes that we have the willpower to use energy productively. Let's dive deep into this energy.

Tuning and understanding your Spiritual Energy will serve you your entire life. I first discovered this truth when my mom's health was deteriorating. I wanted to understand the disease and learn new ways to help my mom manage it. I studied various healing modalities, including reiki, and used these tools with my parents. After every session, my mom would always rave that she felt better, saying she felt relaxed and had this peace of mind. She often referred to me as having healing hands. I also noticed a shift for both Mom and Dad. It was beautiful to watch, and a gift to experience with them. At the time, I didn't fully understand what I was doing. I simply stayed open to the possibility of asking God to use love and light through me to heal them. It wasn't me doing the work, I simply was inviting God to use me as the vessel to help my parents.

To this day, I still utilize and use focused energy to heal myself, others, and even animals. My dog Lexi, loves when I use frankincense essential oil on her and give her reiki treatments! There have been times when she's had symptoms in the past that, even after several tests and an expensive vet bill, they still had no clue what she had or the cause. I decided to use the oil on her and move energy towards her, and within minutes, I noticed a shift and a deeper connection with her.

It was powerful, supernatural, and amazing to offer this gift to her. I continue to use this technique to this day, whenever she's having an "off" day.

Know Your Starting Point!

Visit your physician or health care professional and complete a whole-body health assessment in order to find your starting point. This will include blood work and a complete physical checkup so that you address any deficiencies or anything that needs to be addressed immediately. I love the prevention approach as opposed to waiting for signs of symptoms to happen before we decide to visit a physician. Often, one's minerals are depleted, and if we know our starting point, then we don't need to guess. We can provide the proper care that our bodies need.

Stress plays a key role in your health and wellbeing, and when you're stressed, your body ends up using your reserves, depleting you. Knowing what your body needs, aside from the obvious necessities of rest, food, and water, is important so you begin to move from survival mode into the thriving mode of living. This will help you with creating your best health care plan.

We spoke about compassion fatigue in our last chapter. What are some tools you can use to minimize this fatigue within you? Some forms of health care treatment for my clients (which I personally use as well) include:

- ♥ Massage therapy
- ♥ Yoga

- 💜 Pilates
- 💜 Acupuncture
- 💜 Ayurvedic techniques
- 💜 Aromatherapy
- 💜 Physiotherapy
- 💜 Reiki
- 💜 Baths and spas
- 💜 Mindfulness practice
- 💜 Prayer and meditation
- 💜 Joining a caregiver support group
- 💜 Cognitive therapy
- 💜 Coaching and mentor programs
- 💜 Exercise

Bottom line, engage in activities that will make you feel healthier and vibrant!

One of my favorite techniques is mindfulness. You can do this anywhere and anytime. What is mindfulness meditation? This means being one-hundred percent in what you're presently doing—not thinking about anything else and really sensing, feeling, observing the present moment. This is actually the greatest gift you can offer to someone else, including yourself—to fully experience and *be* in the *now*. Give your full attention, mind, heart, and spirit to their presence. To do this, one must stop, breathe, and be curious about what they hear, smell, taste, and see. Listen in and tune in to the beauty of life. This alone has brought me peace of mind many times when I was experiencing anxiety, worry, or fear. I teach this technique to my clients so that they too can experience peace of mind, calmness, and joy in their hearts. These are moments when grace comes in. Grace flows through us when we invite her in. It's like consciously inviting her into our home. In this example, our home is our soul and our heart.

The psychological and physical impact the caregiver role had on me and my loved ones was a daily management pursuit. During the difficult times, I've often reframed my thinking to focus on being grateful. I was given the opportunity and called to be a caregiver. What a sacred and precious gift. The time spent with my parents deepened my relationship with them before they died and transitioned over. The beauty in all of this is that they are still alive and present in my heart. I cherish those beautiful moments we shared together and the intimacy we experienced through heartfelt discussions. It's been said that we often don't remember what people do, but we certainly remember how they made us feel. Those moments of love are like diamonds, so rare and luminous.

Managing Your Boundaries

Managing your boundaries with different energy tools includes connecting with your Spirit and self. There's more to you, so much more, than your physical body. As you learn new ways to move energy, discharge blocks and negative energy, you start loving yourself more. The good news is that when you discover your block, you can release it and be free.

An effective way you can release your energy blocks is using a technique called Emotional Freedom Technique (EFT tapping). We have twelve major meridian points in our body that correspond to an internal organ, however EFT mainly focuses on nine points:

- ♥ karate chop (KC): small intestine meridian
- ♥ top of head (TH): governing vessel
- ♥ eyebrow (EB): bladder meridian
- ♥ side of the eye (SE): gallbladder meridian
- ♥ under the eye (UE): stomach meridian
- ♥ under the nose (UN): governing vessel
- ♥ chin (Ch): central vessel
- ♥ beginning of the collarbone (CB): kidney meridian
- ♥ under the arm (UA): spleen meridian

Before commencing the healing technique, you want to identify only one issue, usually a feeling or pain you have. For example, I'm sad my mother is not well. After you identify your problem area, you need to set a benchmark level of intensity. The intensity level is rated on a scale from zero to ten with ten being the worst or most difficult. The scale assesses the emotional or physical pain and discomfort you feel from your focal issue. Prior to tapping, you need to establish a phrase that explains what you're trying to address. It must focus on two main goals:

- ♥ acknowledging the issues
- ♥ accepting yourself despite the problem

The common setup phrase is: "Even though I have this [fear or problem], I deeply and completely accept myself." For example, if we continue using the issue noted above, you will say: "Even though I'm sad my mother is not well, I deeply and completely accept myself." This is the phrase you will be saying at each tapping point and you will repeat the following sequence two or three times.

Now, begin by tapping the karate chop point while simultaneously reciting your setup phrase three times. Then, tap each following point seven times, moving down the body in this order:

- ❤ eyebrow
- ❤ side of the eye
- ❤ under the eye
- ❤ under the nose
- ❤ chin
- ❤ beginning of the collarbone
- ❤ under the arm

Remember, while tapping each point, you want to repeat out loud the issue you are experiencing, "Even though I'm sad my mother is unwell, I deeply and completely accept myself." At the end of your sequence, rate your intensity level on a scale from zero to ten. Compare your results with your initial intensity level. If you haven't reached zero, repeat this process until you do.

Aroma Radiant Technique (ART)

Here's another technique, I call ART, which I love using on myself and with my clients. The Aroma Radiant Technique is a simple process designed to help you get from where you are to where you want to be. For example, you may feel stuck, confused, exhausted, overwhelmed or have goals and feel hopeless about ever reaching them, especially when your focus is on caring for your loved one.

In the moments when you feel anxious, overwhelmed, or your energy is low, use essential oils and this technique to change your state. (Note: make sure you get oils from a trusted source—one that owns their own farms and distilleries and manages the quality process from beginning to end. Inferior oils can be toxic and need to be avoided.)

First: Set an intention, creating a sentence in the present tense. Here's an example: "I have harmonious relationships." Write down your intention. Say the intention out loud and notice the distracting thoughts that come up. Common thoughts that may come up: That's not possible. You're tired. You have no idea how to do that. You have tried that before and you failed. This won't work. Override these thoughts with your intention.

Second: Now, tune into your body and notice where you're feeling this negative feeling. Become aware of the feeling and where you feel it in your body. Drift into an earlier time, a memory, where you've felt the same feeling. Close your eyes. Focus on the memory, the feeling, the negative thought and the sensation in your body while smelling the essential oil that you feel attracted to, (choosing specific oils are personal and your body knows what aromas you're attracted to and what your body needs). The "go to" oils I use often for this technique are frankincense and lavender.

Third: Allow feelings to just pass through you as you smell the oil. Feelings are like waves and no wave lasts forever. See what happens to the image and feelings in your body. Notice your thoughts. Revisit your intention and say it out loud, three times. "I have harmonious relationships." You will experience a shift.

Fourth: Now create an affirmation that expresses the new, positive belief and attitude you wish to install. The affirmation should be in the present tense, positive and to the point, such as: "I am organized, efficient, and friendly with my dad's health care team." Say your affirmation with confidence and enthusiasm. Repeat the affirmation for two minutes, morning and night, while standing in your favorite power pose. Once you've said your affirmation, you will be in a good mental state to tackle what needs to be done today. Experiment with this technique for thirty days and notice the change.

As a caregiver, you have to learn ways to be self-compassionate. Every day, do something for yourself. This needs to be your daily goal. The rhythm of a caregiver is to fill up with life-giving energy, give to others, and then refill. Every day, it's important to schedule this in your calendar and make this part of your morning and/or evening routine. Whatever works best for you is perfect. Simply make it work for you and do this as a priority like brushing your teeth!

These tools and techniques are not exclusive to caregivers. You can lead by example and help your loved ones create a self-care plan for themselves. Teach them ways to meditate and ways to care for themselves. Passing it forward will serve both of you in the long run. It also helps create a stronger bond between you. You can share about your experiences and help each other grow stronger connecting with Spirit and self.

When you show up for your loved one, you will show up with more compassion and patience. There will be a calmness about you that prepares you for any adversity coming your way. This doesn't exclude any challenges coming your way, this simply prepares you to be resilient when life happens.

Let's do something together right now. Close your eyes and focus on your breath. Just breathe deeply. Now breathe in for a count of five, pause for three, and exhale for a count of five. Do this three times. This helps you slow down and helps your nervous system relax. It helps you feel more energy entering your body and you become more aware of your body. Simply notice what you're noticing without any judgement. When thoughts come up, simply allow them to pass along. The goal is not to get rid of thoughts but to become aware of them with gentle mindfulness. If this is new to you, you will think that you can't meditate because you have a busy mind. This is simply not true. Everyone has the power to meditate, and this is a skill that can be learned too. What's actually happening, perhaps for the first time, is that you're noticing your thoughts. You never really paid attention to them before, you just thought. Now you are observing your thinking. When you notice your mind wandering, simply bring your attention back to your next breath.

Also, you want to breathe into your abdomen. Society has learned to breathe into their chest; however, let's go back to the beginning when you were a baby. Babies breathe into their belly. Their bellies rise and lower with each breath. Notice your belly fill up, and if it helps, place your hands over your abdomen, close your eyes, and breathe. Do this exercise several times a day or as often as you need to, to relax your mind and body and slow down. There have been numerous scientific research studies on the benefits of mindfulness and meditation techniques for your health and wellbeing. When challenges come up and you don't know what to say or do, focus on your breath, and just breathe deeply, for a count of five. This will help you take your next bold action step.

You can't rush through a loved one's care. You have to slow down. Be present. Be grateful. Now. This is a rare opportunity to be your loved one's caregiver. So don't miss it!

Chapter 8

STEP 5—HOW DO I CARE FOR MYSELF AND BE GUILT-FREE?

am the most important person in my life. When I first read this statement, I felt really uncomfortable. I didn't know at the time why. "There's no way this can be true," I thought. I certainly knew this wasn't the way I was brought up, to think that I was the most important person. *Everyone else comes first* is what I was taught. Thinking the opposite brought up feelings of selfishness, self-centeredness, thoughts of unworthiness, and that I don't deserve loving myself first. These thoughts are absolutely false and, I might add, ridiculous when you read them.

You are here on earth for a purpose. Each and every one of us are so unique and can never be duplicated exactly the same. We are all individual snowflakes with a unique blueprint. When we recognize our own value and worth, we have more to offer others. When we love ourselves deeply, we can love others deeply. You are not capable of loving another if you don't love yourself first. I invite you to write this statement on a sticky note, in fact, write on eight sticky notes the same message: "I am the most important person in my life." Post them everywhere. I assure you when you start reading these words and seeing them consistently, you start believing them, and something inside of you shifts. The most beautiful transformation occurs. You become empowered with your own light and beauty. You start appreciating yourself more and you start creating necessary boundaries and learning to say no, with ease and grace.

Find ways to care for yourself first and make yourself a priority. Taking this one step further, I encourage you to look in the mirror, look into your eyes, and say these words to yourself, "I love you." At first, this will feel awkward and likely uncomfortable. Do it anyway. Look at yourself in the mirror, and instead of judging or criticizing, simply tell yourself, "I love you." If this is difficult for you, get a picture of yourself from when you were around six or seven years old, pin it up in your bathroom, and start talking to her, teaching her how to take care of herself. Simply look at the picture and start talking to her. You could literally say, "Good morning. I love you." Create a relationship with the part of yourself that might feel vulnerable and who really needs you to care deeply for her. Now, this won't work for you if you only say it once or twice. I invite you to do an experiment, saying this every day, twice a day, or even better, every time you walk by a mirror or stand in front of a mirror, say out loud while looking deeply into your eyes, "I love you."

One of my mentors shared this activity with me once, and my first reaction was, "That's not going to work for me!" I had thoughts that weren't serving me and my wellbeing. I had these thoughts and did the activity anyway. The first few times, it felt strange, and I could see the discomfort in my face. Then one day, my energy shifted. When I looked in the mirror, this light came through my eyes, and this joy entered my body. I had this sense of appreciation and love for the person I was looking at. My eyes lit up and a big smile came over my face. I remember this same feeling when I delivered my next-door neighbor's baby in her home. I held this newborn baby in my arms and was amazed at the miracle and gift that I was holding. Just writing this out and reminding myself of this beautiful gift of life and honor of serving this mother and child, still lights me up and brings me tears of joy to this day. This event happened in 2006, and the feeling is still as pure and loving and joyful now as it was on that cold February winter day.

There is nothing to feel guilty about for loving yourself and caring for yourself deeply. This needs to be a priority. Otherwise, you will seek things and people outside of yourself that will give you temporary feelings of love and security, all while looking for love in all the wrong places to fulfill yourself. Growing up as a caregiver for my mom was both a gift and a challenge. She was diagnosed with an autoimmune disease when I was six years old, and by the time I was eight years old, I was going to the grocery store, buying groceries, cleaning, cooking, and taking care of my mom. At the time, I can assure you I wasn't thinking this was a gift. I wanted someone to care for me. Who was taking care of me? I didn't feel loved, and at some point, I started to become angry that I had to stand up for myself and demand that I play outside with my friends. That turned into looking for love in all the wrong places.

We create this emotional hunger that disconnects us from our true self, and entangles us in roles and responsibilities that we've come to believe is the truth of us, such as we were born to be a caregiver. This childhood pattern continues until we bring conscious light to the pattern. We are unable to discern at an early age, whether the patterns we take on will benefit us in this lifetime or not. Whether they are rooted in love or fear. Whether they will help expand or contract our true self. We are meant for more. Our patterns and history don't define us. They shape us, but they don't define who we become. We define ourselves by the choices we make, and the actions we take.

You are a gift to the world. Regardless of the behaviors, experiences, feelings of self-doubt and unworthiness, traumas, conditions, circumstances, or the situation you've been raised in. You are a luminous light being. The world needs you to shine your light outwardly, and most importantly, to invite the light inwardly. When we are healed, then we can easily tune into the power and heal others too. This is one of the most beautiful, magnificent gifts the world has ever received! The ability to heal oneself and others, through love and light. Again, I emphasize, if you don't take care of your own happiness first, how can you take care of anyone else's? Make it a priority! And if you need help, I'm here to help you. My intention is to help you see your own light and magnificence while you're caring for others. It's about creating both/ and scenarios in your life. Caring for a loved one doesn't mean forgetting or delaying caring about yourself. I used to think this way until I stopped this limited thinking and found ways to create yes/and situations, which I'm sharing with you in this book and through The Graceful Process.

I am here to help you understand the truth about who you are. You are an energetic being. Your thoughts, your feelings, your actions, are energy. It is a scientific fact that we all have the capability to heal every cell in our body. The best way to understand this is shared by a cellular biologist, Bruce Lipton. He has been discovering that our bodies are made up of trillions of cells. We are a community of trillions of cells. What we think and feel is the control center and we are the leaders of this control center, our community of cells. If you are encouraging, inspiring, and work with your people, they will respond accordingly. If you are mean and send your people negative thoughts and don't work with them, they will become rebellious and won't work in coherence with you.

Our bodies do the same thing. Our cells respond to consciousness and to the environment they are in. Our current medical system is based on the mentality that the genes we are born with are a read-only file and can't be changed. This is false. Our cells are constantly changing, and we can cultivate health through our lifestyle choices. Our thoughts create our feelings, and our feelings get imprinted into our bodies through our nervous systems. Therefore, if we become mindful and notice our thoughts and feelings, we have the power to change our inner and outer environment. This is a skill that can be learned and must be learned to live a life of joy and grace.

When you're not feeling well or you're having negative thoughts, what do you do? You become the observer. You pause that thought. Ask yourself *what am I feeling right now?* Notice what you're noticing. And reframe that thought. Train your mind to look for the good in everything. At first, it will feel awkward because it's new and when things are new, it's foreign to us. It's like learning a new language. The best way to learn a new language is to immerse yourself in the culture. Therefore, I encourage you to immerse yourself in the culture. Surround yourself with others who are uplifting and who believe in you, inspire you, and see your true beauty and magnificence. Just being around these people will influence your feelings and thoughts. Learn to sit with feelings of joy and appreciation so that you become used to those feelings. Another way of doing this is by recalling a time where you've felt really good, inspired, and loved, and create that feeling again in your body similar to the way I recalled delivering my neighbor's baby into the world. We are working on a cellular level in your mind, body, and spirit. This will create a new emotional blueprint in your nervous system.

Managing Your Feelings

Self-esteem is how I feel about myself, therefore how I treat myself, therefore how I behave. When I share with others that I'm a recovering addict, they react and ask me what I was addicted to. It's not about what I was addicted to; it's about becoming aware of why I would choose something outside of myself to fix how I feel while also harming myself.

Addiction isn't about the drug of choice. It's about outsourcing one's emotional process into something else and it backfires. The reality is I was very defensive about being seen—I mean really being seen. I stumbled into a twelve-step program that helped me see myself and others like me. It's an amazing feeling to see and feel the transformation when we recognize we're not alone, seek help, and are vulnerable about who we are.

As caregivers, it's normal that we run on empty because, as a child, we usually learn this through family dynamics and behaviors. It's normal that caregivers stay in this role as givers. An emotional shock absorber, we say, "Don't worry about me. I'll be alright. Let's worry about you." And we always redirect the topic of conversation to others instead of sharing what's really going on within us.

Let's look at your ability to receive. What's your ability to say no? What's your ability to say that you need help? What's your ability to have self-respect and look after yourself and therefore give generously from a place of abundance, rather than giving from a place that is running on empty? There's no point in only telling you techniques for coping with your loved one. Unless you get comfortable in your own shoes, you have self-respect, and you maintain that respect for yourself, you will always run on empty.

What are the feelings that you're experiencing? And "okay" and "fine" aren't feelings. Some of us have been programmed to not feel at all and to not show emotions because it's a sign of weakness. We don't let others know what we're feeling because we'll lose the deal. Some of us, due to our professions, have been trained to stay strong for the purpose of work and not share our feelings with others. Regardless of the reasons, if you know the feelings you are feeling, then you have a chance to take responsibility and represent yourself in the world with dignity and respect.

Affirmindset

So we've learned that feelings come from our thoughts. Therefore, let's look at the thoughts that you have and ask yourself, "Do I have a healthy mindset?" Here are some thoughts that caregivers have shared with me:

- ❤ I'm not good enough.
- ❤ I feel guilty.
- ❤ I'm not worthy.
- ❤ What's wrong with me?
- ❤ I was born to take care of my parents.
- ❤ Nobody understands what I'm going through.
- ❤ I'm all alone.
- ❤ It's not the right time to care for me.
- ❤ I don't deserve…
- ❤ I'm not a priority.

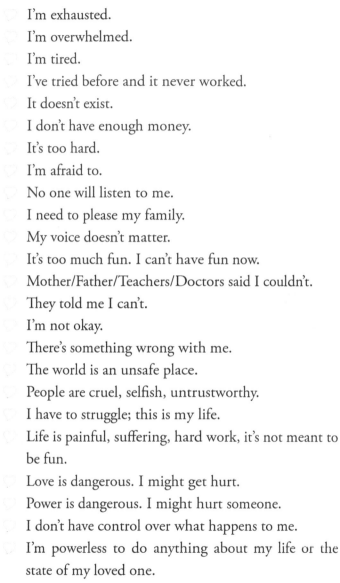

I'm exhausted.

I'm overwhelmed.

I'm tired.

I've tried before and it never worked.

It doesn't exist.

I don't have enough money.

It's too hard.

I'm afraid to.

No one will listen to me.

I need to please my family.

My voice doesn't matter.

It's too much fun. I can't have fun now.

Mother/Father/Teachers/Doctors said I couldn't.

They told me I can't.

I'm not okay.

There's something wrong with me.

The world is an unsafe place.

People are cruel, selfish, untrustworthy.

I have to struggle; this is my life.

Life is painful, suffering, hard work, it's not meant to be fun.

Love is dangerous. I might get hurt.

Power is dangerous. I might hurt someone.

I don't have control over what happens to me.

I'm powerless to do anything about my life or the state of my loved one.

Realize that these thinking programs and negative beliefs are only beliefs! They have no objective truth. The most powerful action you can do is to change your own beliefs about yourself, the nature of life, people, and reality, to something more positive, and become that person. Delete and clear old programming and replace with new and *Affirmindset*. Here are some new beliefs from *The Creative Visualization Workbook* by Shakti Gawain:

- ❤ I now release my entire past.
- ❤ It is complete, and I am free!
- ❤ I now dissolve all negative, limiting beliefs. They have no power over me!
- ❤ I now forgive and release everyone in my life. We are all happy and free.
- ❤ I don't have to try to please others. I am naturally loveable and likeable no matter what I do!
- ❤ I now let go of all accumulated guilt, fears, resentment, disappointment, and grudges. I am free and clear!
- ❤ All of my negative self-images and attitudes are now dissolved. I love and appreciate myself!
- ❤ All barriers to my full expression and enjoyment of life are now dissolved.
- ❤ The world is a beautiful place to be.
- ❤ The Universe always provides.
- ❤ I am willing to be my true, magnificent self.
- ❤ Every day I am growing more beautiful and more radiantly healthy!
- ❤ Everything I do adds to my health and beauty.
- ❤ Everything I eat adds to my health, beauty, and attractiveness.

♥ I am good to my body, and my body is good to me.

♥ I am now vibrant, strong, and in perfect health no matter what I do.

I am growing stronger and more powerful every day.

I now desire to eat only those things that are best for me at any given time.

The more I love and appreciate myself, the more beautiful I am becoming.

♥ I am now irresistibly attractive to others.

As well, here are some favorite Affirmindset mantras I use:

♥ I am committed to being the best version of myself every day.

I pamper myself on a weekly basis, receiving body-work and rest that rejuvenates my body and soul.

I have restful sleeps and wake up refreshed and recharged.

I am bringing my very best to all my relationship interactions.

I am a transmitter of love and positive energy.

Notice what you're feeling when you say the new beliefs. As mentioned earlier, at first it may feel awkward saying this out loud, and you may not believe them at first. However, I invite you to try this experiment for thirty days. You don't have to be extreme. Just consistent.

Sleep

Enjoy a mental timeout from the rigors of the day, also known as a "brain shutdown." Some may even choose meditation instead of a nap. Studies have shown fifteen to twenty minutes is perfect; otherwise, too much sleep can disrupt your sleep at night. The sweet spot for a power nap according to the Mediterraneans (siesta time) is after lunch and before 3:00 p.m. Anything after 3:00 p.m. could affect your night's sleep.

I also want to emphasize the importance of restorative sleep. How deeply you sleep is vital to brain health, and restorative sleep helps your body heal. When you're asleep, your body is still working on your behalf. Sleeping for seven to eight hours a night, as well as going to bed and waking up at the same time, will improve your health and quality of life. When you don't sleep well and if this extends for a long period of time, you will have symptoms that may impact the homeostasis of your body and cause dis-ease.

Hydration

Drinking enough pure and simple water every day is vital to your health and well-being. No tissue, organ, or gland can function properly without ample supply of this natural fluid. Water is the lifeblood of our existence, second only to air. Without it, we wouldn't survive for long. The most important thing you can do for your health is to drink more water. Many people believe that if we don't feel thirsty, we don't need more water. Nothing could be further from the truth. By the time we feel thirst, we're already quite dehydrated. Try drinking a full glass before you start your day in the morning and a full glass an hour after dinner. Replace sugary soft drinks with water to reduce your calorie intake and to keep caffeine from emptying your body of the water it already has. Get in the habit of taking water with you wherever you go. Drink more often; you will likely find your body feeling better and craving the higher water intake.

Movement

Keep moving your body. New studies have linked diseases to sedentary lifestyles. Daily movement helps combat fatigue and restore energy levels. Get up and move every hour. Take a stroll after eating lunch. Carve out movement-based leisure time and connection time with other people. Health increases with intentionally moving your body. Go for walks with your loved one. My parents enjoyed our daily walks, and it was a great opportunity to deepen our relationship and enjoy quality time together.

As well, you can prevent chronic stress through movement. Our bodies are meant to move and when we're not moving, muscles and joints get stiff. Focus on relaxing and loosening things up. Be sure to take deep breaths in, exhale slowly and move, twist, do side bends, arm and neck stretches. Stretches are highly beneficial and we can do them anywhere, while sitting, standing or lying down. It's important to stretch your muscles out. Find a routine that you enjoy and move.

When we don't move, we don't bring nutrients to our muscles and our joints. We don't get the oxygen flowing, and that is what is going to keep all our systems healthy.

Getting up and walking will help our gastrointestinal system. Nothing will work well if we're stagnant. Remember, movement is super important to maintain our health.

Nutrition

While caring for my parents, I studied the effects of food and nutrition on our bodies. Often, people think that if they take vitamins and minerals and skip meals throughout the day, that this is good for them. I've had clients share some of their meals with me and then wonder why they're not feeling well. Your eating habits and lack of sleep impact your digestion and mineral/vitamin absorption in your body. Eat foods that are life-giving, like fruits, vegetables, beans, etc. There really isn't a best diet, every body is different and everyone's needs are different. You must experiment on your own and find a nutrition plan that works best for you. I strongly suggest you become curious and look into the ingredients of the food you eat. You will be surprised at how many ingredients you can't even pronounce! I have a rule: if I can't pronounce or don't know what's in the food I eat, I simply stay away and don't take that risk. The right nutrition can help you get the most out of life!

When you're exhausted, you're bound to make bad decisions due to fatigue, fear, and panic. Adopt these new habits, and build a vibrant, powerful *Affirmindset* that will lead you to personal growth and caregiving success!

Chapter 9:

STEP 6—HOW CAN I FEEL JOY DURING THIS DIFFICULT TIME?

"There are only two ways to live your life.
One is as though nothing is a miracle.
The other as though everything is a miracle."
- Albert Einstein

D o you know the difference between happiness and joy? Happiness is a fleeting state, a temporary high. On the other hand, joy is an always present state of being. Joy is a fundamental energy that lifts us up and exists within us. Joy is part of our nature and our birthright. We tend to get caught up with the busyness of the day, caring for others, working, and we're not making joy a priority. Why not take essential steps towards joyful living and bring it everywhere you go?

Just today, I had a friend come over, and he decided to climb a ladder and slide down the slide outside, being playful and joyful. You may think joy is when you see kids playing and that only they can experience joy. Joy can fill anyone's heart at any age! Look at my sixty-year-old neighbor who decided today was the day he was going down that slide! Made us both laugh!

Joyful Meditations

Surround yourself with people that have joy in their hearts. You walk into a room, and there are people who have good vibes and positive energy. The exchange of vibrant energy is so powerful. Hug them! I know this may sound strange, but hugging really helps. In a study on fears and self-esteem published in the journal Psychological Science, research revealed that hugs and touch significantly reduce worry of mortality. Hugs release oxytocin, often called the "love hormone." When people hug or kiss a loved one, oxytocin levels increase. Why not add more love in your life? Make it a point to hug your loved ones daily.

Embrace nature. Nature is the perfect teacher, so be a part of nature. Observe nature, go for long walks, and do walking meditations listening to positive affirmations playing in the background. Be in awe with the beauty of nature. I'm always in complete bliss when I watch a sunrise or a sunset, and I love going for walks with my dog Lexi, who always brings me joy and makes me laugh. The key is to realize that joy is an inner state. Joy lives within you, and joy is not dependent on your external circumstances. Joy loves to share its joy! Bring more joy into your life.

Sense the beauty around you. Notice the details of plants, birds, trees, bugs. This week, get up early and take a few moments of solitude and silence to start your day. Joy arises in those moments of silence, and you'll find the rest of your day is more peaceful. I start each morning with a morning ritual of silence and setting an intention for the day. I set an intention of who I want to "be" and choose thoughts, behaviors, and actions that align with who I want to be. Bringing more joy into your life means you will feel more energy and vitality. Joy gives you direct access to your creativity. It helps you connect with others and with life itself. In fact, when you're in joy, you don't feel lonely or isolated. Being in the state of joy is a meaningful habit you must cultivate. Get started on creating a relationship with joy!

As a gift, I would love to send you a link for a joyful meditation. Send an email to info@josephinegracecoaching.com to receive your copy.

Sacred Spaces

Create soothing spaces in your home. Remove any items that no longer serve you and bring you joy. This action clears space in your home, your mind, and your heart. It creates a soothing environment to live in and helps you appreciate your space even more. Imagine what it would feel like if you surrounded yourself daily *only* with things you loved—from your tea mug to your comfortable bed. How different would you feel? How much joy would enter your life on a daily basis? Clear the clutter, clear your closet, clear paper that you don't need any longer, and donate or give items away to others. Organize your home, car, and then help your loved ones do the same. I remember when my parents moved into a long-term care home and we began the difficult process of sifting through all their items. The good news is they had the opportunity to choose the items that brought them joy and had meaning for them, and all else was either sold or given away. There was freedom in releasing the old for the new beginnings that were happening in their lives.

Gratitude

Appreciate what is around you and in you. Plenty has been written in the last few years about gratitude practices and their benefits. I've seen it transform my life and many of my friends' and clients' lives. I've assigned clients I've worked with a gratitude practice each night where they say and write three things they're most grateful for in their lives. I used to practice this with my parents. I made it a point when I spoke with them to share at least one thing that uplifted their spirit. I also encouraged them to write in a journal the things that had gone well each day, regardless of stress, conditions, or circumstances. Surely, they could find something to be grateful for, and they always did. At first, it was unusual, and so I helped them by pointing things out for them. *The sun is shin-*

ing today. You woke up this morning. We shared a lovely lunch together. We have another opportunity to be together. You have peace in your heart. God loves you, and so do I. I still have my mom's journal that I cherish.

I invite you to do another experiment for seven days. I feel confident that you'll find more joy in every day than you possibly could have imagined simply by being present to what surrounds you and seeing the beauty in everything you see. Remember, when joy arises in you and fills you up, tell yourself: *I deserve to be happy. I deserve to be joyful. I deserve to love my life.* Follow that with, *I am happy, I am joyful, and I love my life.* I'm always in awe of how magnificent my body is, how grateful I am that it supports me every day, and how wonderful that it knows exactly how to heal itself when I provide it with the right support it needs. Our bodies are magnificent machines that speak to us all the time. The question is, are we listening? I encourage you to listen to your body and be curious; find the ways that support your body. Be grateful for your beautiful temple, also known as your body, and fall in love with yourself. Naturally, by appreciating your own body, you will create more energy and vibrancy, and in turn, your energy will pour out onto others.

Gratitude Practice

At the end of the day, just before you fall asleep, sit in a sacred space you've created and make yourself comfortable. Relax.

Think of the day that's coming to an end and choose something you are grateful for (a smile, a new friend, a bird flying by, a phone call, an opportunity, or simply grateful to relax in your bed after a difficult day). Recall the situation in as much detail as possible and feel your gratitude wholeheartedly.

Next, let go of the situation, but stay with the feeling of joyful gratitude as you dive deeper into the feeling itself. This is the joy vibration. By practicing how to connect with this vibration, you will be able to bring joy up within you at any time and in any situation you're in. It takes practice, but be kind to yourself and be consistent. This joy will rise up and shine.

Laughter

It is said that laughter cures. Make a list of all the things that make you laugh. Ask your loved ones the same question. In fact, make a list of all the things that bring you joy as well, and when you're feeling low, look at your list and do one of those things that will lift you up again. Now, I'm not suggesting you don't feel the sadness or other low feelings or that you avoid them. It's absolutely vital for your wellbeing that you experience the ebb and flow of feelings! In uncomfortable and difficult situations, it is very important that you fully meet and embrace what you're experiencing before you proactively dive into joy. We are naturally drawn towards pleasure and comfort rather than pain and discomfort. It can be tempting to use joy as an escape from less comfortable experiences such as sadness, anger, or anything else that you'd prefer not to feel and not to experience. I know this well. I did it for years. You simply don't want to stay in those feelings for a long time. Acknowledge and give the experience the awareness and attention it needs; then, accept and release the feeling.

Watch a comedy. Go to a live comedy. Call a friend who you can count on to always make you laugh. By the way, joy doesn't come from your mind. You can't think your way into joy. It is something you can only feel, sense, live, be. Like any relationship along the way, it will be changing, expanding, and transforming. You will begin to experience joy in new ways—and it will show you who you are in new ways. Develop a strong, living relationship with joy to enjoy a vibrant and fulfilled life. Making joy a priority in your life is essential. Go ahead and give yourself permission to make joy one of the highest priorities in your life!

Chapter 10:

STEP 7—AM I MAKING DECISIONS FROM LOVE OR FEAR?

You've learned about "joy frequency" in the previous chapter, and you may be wondering what on earth do vibrations and frequencies have to do with love and fear? Well, I'm glad you asked. There are many fabulous scientists, doctors, and teachers out there who can absolutely dive into the scientific facts about vibrations and frequencies. I'm going to do my best to simplify it for you. Imagine yourself walking into a room where a couple has just finished arguing. You don't hear them say a word when you enter the room; however, you can feel the tension and the negative vibes from the argument that just occurred. Their bodies have energy that transmits a frequency, a vibration, that ripples into those around them and into the ether. It has a lasting impact and effect. All of a sudden, if you're not aware, you can pick up these energies and walk around with them instead of simply observing, detaching, and moving forward.

Love and fear have frequencies and vibrations too. In fact, all feelings and emotions are in the energy field. I recently read an article by Dr. Shirley Marshall who stated, "When we live in the love vibration, our energy resonates at a high frequency, and we express the God-qualities of compassion, forgiveness, tolerance, respect, generosity, joy, peace—all that inspires, empowers and enhances life. The love vibration lifts us to a higher state of consciousness and frees us of the thoughts, feelings, and actions that minimize and victimize us." Therefore, when you are making decisions for yourself and your loved one, are you choosing the best decision, the decision that comes from love?

An example would be your loved one receives a cancer diagnosis, yet they're not experiencing any symptoms, only a diagnosis that was given due to a regular physical check-up based on a small lump they discovered. Instead of being curious and gathering second and third opinions, they decide, out of fear, that they want to go ahead and have surgery and remove the cancer. This decision was based out of fear. Another option, out of love, would be coming from compassion and staying open to the possibility of healing and hope. I'm not suggesting not to have surgery. I'm simply suggesting staying open to possibilities and opportunities to see things in a new light.

Our best decisions and experiences come from love, an expansive feeling where you can physically feel your body opening up. Making decisions out of love results in peace of mind and an open heart. On the other hand, fear has a contractive feeling, restricts flow in your body, and causes anxiety, keeping you in survival mode. Love is the highest vibration. Love is an action. Choose love.

The best and simplest explanation I've found that has helped me the most is the definition of love in Corinthians: "Love is patient. Love is kind. It always protects, always trusts, always hopes, always perseveres. Love never fails." When our actions, behaviors, and words are aligned with this definition, then we can be assured that we are making decisions out of love. These actions expand more love into your relationships, your family's lives, and ripple forward into the world. In the moment of deciding, pause and ask yourself, *Is what I'm saying or doing kind, patient, hopeful, and trusting?* If the answer is yes, proceed forward and do or say out of love. If you realize that it's the opposite—impatient, fearful, giving up, mean, hopeless—then you know that this is out of fear. Love is expansive, and fear is contractive.

How to generate a state of love goes back to your thoughts. What thoughts do you need to think that will cause you to feel love? Love is the most powerful force in the universe. Love can heal. Love can create abundance. Love is the path to living an inspired life. Love forgives faults and imperfections. Love says, "You can do it. Let me tell you how *amazing* you are." Love listens. Love inspires. Choose love. One of the quickest ways to tune into love is to focus on what you appreciate in others. Give thanks for all the things that are going *right* in your life. Stop dwelling on the things that are going wrong for you. Bring into your awareness all that is awesome – like your health, the roof over your head, the warm and comfy bed you sleep in, your friends, family, and pets. Make a decision to sustain a state of love by focusing on loving thoughts and actions.

Make a Lasting Change

Dr. Joe Dispenza's work has been a breakthrough for thousands of people, including myself. He details how you can rewire your brain, recondition your body, and make a lasting change. He goes into the science and neurology of the brain and how it works. I love his work and encourage you to study it too. I also appreciate how he explains the new field of biology work on epigenetics, that the environment influences the behavior of cells without changing the genetic codes. He asserts that it's energy that is the vital force that controls life.

What can cause disease? A disruption in the signal to the brain not allowing the body to function. There are only three ways to mess up the signal: trauma, toxins (chemistry), and thought (mind). Therefore, if you change your mind, you can change your biology. The brain is what controls the signal and controls the cells in your body. Therefore, you control the genes; the genes do not control you. How is it that in a family you have parents who have or had a disease, and only one or none of the kids develop the symptoms and disease as the parents? If you solely focus on genes and the theory that once your parents have it, you will have the same disease because of your genes, then you will step into this blueprint and live out of fear.

I've seen this happen too often. A client in her forties was told by a physician that since her parent has cancer, there's a very good chance she will develop cancer. Therefore, it's best to take an HPV vaccine to prevent cancer. My client displayed no signs of symptoms and refused the treatment after she did some research and realized there were other ways to build her immune system and do her best to prevent cancer. Everyone has their own choices to make. Receiving a diagnosis and prognosis can be very difficult to hear. One day your life is "normal," and the next, your life changes. It's important to do your own research and become empowered with knowledge and, most importantly, to make decisions and take action based on love instead of fear.

It's Not about What You Need to Do. It's about Who You Need to Be!

I love experiments! Here's another invitation to experiment with a daily/weekly practice of pointing yourself toward truth—toward the magnificent, valuable, loveable person who is innately resilient, resourceful, and able to respond to any situation from your inner being. I encourage you to choose a frequency/duration you know you can win in.

Tune to recorded affirmations of the truth about yourself. At least once a day, listen to uplifting meditations, pause when challenged to question the negative thought that arises and re-frame any false/limiting beliefs to empowering ones. This will help strengthen your spiritual muscles to care for yourself.

When a low mood or thought comes up, you can pause and recognize *this is just a thought*. Thoughts are not real. When you don't feed it or give it attention, it will pass - like a passing cloud in the sky. Any time you feel low - vibrating at a low frequency - it is not your inner wisdom speaking. It is the old paradigm and programming, the conditioning that is acting out and popping in from time to time. We all have conditioned patterns. As you learn to recognize your patterns, you can invite yourself to not take it so seriously. The truth is, it has nothing to do with your essence, and it can never touch your true self. At some point, you just agreed with these paradigms and then lived according to these paradigm beliefs. It's part of your human experience, but now you have a new level of awareness. You can change your thoughts and feelings and vibrate at a high frequency. Make decisions from love. Always choose love.

Chapter 11:

STEP 8—HOW DO I IMPROVE MY RELATIONSHIPS?

Lord, make me an instrument of your peace.
Where there is hatred, let me bring love.
Where there is offense, let me bring pardon.
Where there is discord, let me bring union.
Where there is error, let me bring truth.
Where there is doubt, let me bring faith.
Where there is despair, let me bring hope.
Where there is darkness, let me bring your light.
Where there is sadness, let me bring joy.
O Master, let me not seek as much
to be consoled as to console,

to be understood as to understand,
to be loved as to love,
for it is in giving that one receives,
it is in self-forgetting that one finds,
it is in pardoning that one is pardoned,
it is in dying that one is raised to eternal life.

This is a popular prayer used by many, and it's become popular through the teachings of St. Francis. The twelve-step program also uses this prayer, along with another prayer: "God, grant me the serenity to accept the things I cannot change, courage to change the things I can, and wisdom to know the difference."

Both of these prayers are high vibrational prayers. They bring meaning, acceptance, and forgiveness. You can use these guidelines to improve your relationships with others. I've spoken to many caregivers whose loved ones had died, and during our conversations, what surfaced was their regret. They regretted not going to visit their loved ones often, not telling their loved one thank you and I love you, not forgiving them for past hurts, not apologizing for something they've done, not appreciating more moments and time with them, not having heart-to-heart conversations with them, not asking them what their wishes were when they died, or not preparing for the inevitable death.

There's one thing that's certain—death will come. I know many are afraid to look death in the face, but death will come anyway. Avoiding it, denying it, and not accepting death will not change the reality of death. However, the good news is that the day hasn't arrived for your loved one. You have an opportunity to not regret the precious time and moments you have with them, to choose love instead of fear as your driving force to care for yourself and for your loved one who counts on you for support.

What can you do to improve your relationship with your loved ones? You can start by taking small steps every day and preparing for a peaceful and graceful journey. You can have the heart-to-heart conversations with your family. Delegate tasks, ask for support, create a schedule and include self-care, set boundaries, and learn to say no. Be in the moment with your loved ones, appreciate the time you have with them, and be prepared. Living in the *now* is healthy and leads to better relationships with your family and health team.

Often, people want to offer support, yet they have no idea what to say or do to help. To receive effective support and improve your relationships, help your loved one identify what they need and don't need. When you ask for help, be able to clearly identify your needs. For many, asking and accepting help can be difficult. But once they do open themselves up to ask for what they need, acknowledge them. If you offer to do something, follow through with it. That simple. Whether you're offering to drive them to a doctor's appointment, do yard work, clean their room, cook a meal, do some grocery shopping - whatever it is, just make sure you follow through.

Some ways to offer support that you can share with others are:

- ❤ Home-cooked meals
- ❤ Help with grooming (pedicure, manicure, makeup, haircuts)
- ❤ Clean the house and help organize their space
- ❤ Do the laundry
- ❤ Go for walks in the park with them
- ❤ Enjoy their favorite ice cream or dessert together
- ❤ Do grocery shopping
- ❤ Join them for a tea
- ❤ Plant flowers in their garden
- ❤ Bring them a plant

I've also heard from several clients and friends that sometimes all they want is a loved one's presence, someone to be there beside them. Even if they're not having a conversation about anything, simply silently enjoying each other's company can be helpful. I found enjoyment in being in my parents' room reading a book while they watched TV. Simply being beside them brought us all peace of mind, and the number one thing I like to do is silently send them good thoughts, love, and light energy. There's never a limit to this act of kindness, and you don't even have to ask them for permission!

I found this list in a book written by Lori Hope, called *Help Me Live*. She shares principles of respectful, caring, and compassionate communication. She calls this list, "Instead of saying that, you might say this." I've chosen a few from her list to share with you.

- ❤ Instead of asking "How's your health?," you might ask: "How are you doing today?" If they say they're okay, say: "I care about you and want to understand how you're feeling. If you don't want to talk now, no worries, but I am ready to listen when and if you do."

♥ Instead of asking "How did it go at the doctor's today?," you might say, "So you went to the doctor today. If you want to talk about it, you know I want to listen."

♥ Instead of asking, "Have you tried this treatment?," you might offer, "If you're interested in hearing about different treatments, let me know, and I'll do some research for you."

♥ Instead of asking, "Are you cured now?," try asserting, "You look terrific. I hope you feel great!"

♥ Instead of saying, "I know how you feel," you could admit, "I'll never know exactly how you feel, but I'll do my best to understand if you want to talk about it."

♥ Instead of saying, "At least they caught it early," practice saying, "I'm sorry you're having to go through this. I'm here for you." (In this instance, I wonder if saying "I'm sorry" is relevant. I realize we as a society use "I'm sorry" too frequently without actually paying attention to the meaning of the words! Saying it with meaning usually admits a wrongdoing and the hurt that was inflicted on the person you're apologizing to. Why do we say, "I'm sorry for your loss," or "I'm sorry that you're going through this?" Consider saying something like, "It's difficult you're having to go through this. I'm here for you.")

♥ My favorite one of all: instead of assuming that your loved one knows how much you love him (her), look him right in the eye and say, "I love you so much. You mean the world to me." Then give them a hug. Instead of saying anything, hold a hand, touch an arm, or offer a hug.

How To Listen

In *The Road Less Travelled*, M. Scott Peck wrote, "True listening, total concentration on the other, is always a manifestation of love." Love never fails and always heals. To help someone without saying a thing, maintain eye contact, keep your mouth closed, and don't interrupt them. Forget yourself in that moment and keep the focus on them. Resist multitasking, limit distractions, don't interrogate, withhold judgment, empathize, and turn off your advice-o-matic. If you're thinking about how to fix someone, you're not listening. If you must offer advice, ask permission first, and be willing to accept a "no, thanks."

Cultivate Relationships

It's interesting. I learned the most important lessons from my mom and dad's journey during their stay in the long-term care home. They were liked by many, and they cultivated relationships with their professional caregivers. It wasn't easy for them to get used to the change of environment when leaving their home. They were moved in and out of hospitals during their terminal phase and had radiation treatments, injections, and several doctors' appointments. Building good personal relationships with people you have to deal with most frequently has a significant impact for both family caregivers and patients, often in the form of more attentive and personalized treatment.

Professional caregivers have a challenging task to give high quality and safe care to your loved one, improve the odds of survival and recovery, and provide empathy and care to every patient, day in and day out. It's the acts of kindness from staff that drew my parents into personal relationships with them. For you, as a devoted and dedicated caregiver, it's important to establish positive and constructive relationships with the professional health care team. Your loved one will be even better served, and you'll find it easier to do your job as an advocate.

Let go of the past hurts and accept that we are all humans who make mistakes. No one is perfect without making mistakes in life. Why hang on to past hurts and regrets? Why not choose to forgive for whatever pain or hurts that were caused in the past? Mother Teresa once said, "If we really want to love, we must learn how to forgive." If someone has hurt you, betrayed you, or broken your heart, find a way to begin the forgiveness process, for this person has helped you learn about trust and the importance of being more discerning about the people you open your heart to.

Researchers have found, holding onto resentment contributes to increased heart disease and weakened immunity and letting go of old grudges reduces stress, anxiety, and depression. People who forgive tend to have better relationships, feel happier and more optimistic, and enjoy greater psychological wellbeing (Deepak Chopra).

I provide a process where my clients make a list of hurts and people/places/things that have caused them pain, and I guide them through to release these pains. Energetically, a shift happens for them and for the others even when the others aren't confronted in person. Holding on to hurts, grudges, and resentments actually energetically blocks your flow and the ability for life to happen through you. When you forgive, you release the block in your body and soul and clear the pathway for love and light to move through you.

This is why I believe St. Francis's prayer is so powerful, and I've seen this prayer transform lives, including my own. When you say these words and really live these words, you become naturally transformed. "Make me an instrument of peace. Where there is darkness, let me bring your light. Where there is sadness, let me bring joy. Where there is despair, let me bring hope. Where there is discord, let me bring union. Where there is hatred, let me bring love. Where there is doubt, let me bring faith. Where there is offense, let me bring pardon. Where there is error, let me bring truth."

> *"Too often we underestimate the power of a touch,*
> *a smile, a kind word, a listening ear, an honest*
> *compliment, or the smallest act of caring, all of which*
> *have the potential to turn a life around."*
> – Leo Buscaglia

Poet and spiritual teacher Maya Angelou said on a radio show, *"I've learned that people will forget what you said, will forget what you did, but people will never forget how you made them feel."*

Connect With Your Higher Self

You may have had glimpses of connecting to your higher self. You've asked yourself a question, and then you receive an "out of the blue" answer. It can come in many different ways: a phone call, an email, someone says something that answers your question, and synchronicities start occurring. These are ways your higher self responds to your question. This is the way Spirit communicates with you and speaks to you. Pay attention and listen.

You may refer to your higher self as communicating with God through prayer. Ask God questions, and be grateful and appreciative when the support you've asked for comes your way. Remember, you're never alone.

Chapter 12:

HOW IN THE WORLD DID I END UP HERE?

Whether you chose to be a caregiver or were suddenly appointed the caregiver's role, you've realized and experienced a shock of some sort when your loved one received the diagnosis. Being diagnosed with a fatal disease is everyone's biggest fear. There's so much information coming from all directions that you may feel overwhelmed, angry, or confused. "Healthy" and "normal" have just disappeared from you and your loved one's life. You may even be in denial and start fantasizing that you'll wake up tomorrow and find out that this was all a bad dream. You may even feel resentful; after all, you didn't sign up to set your own life aside to become a caregiver. You need to learn ways to better handle their care so that you can offer the best support and foster hope.

Your emotions are real, and confronting them is the first step in coming to grips with your caregiver role. You're probably wondering how this unexpected journey will go and how it will end. You may think you're all alone or you're looking for support, guidance, or help. Maybe you are uncertain where to look or even what to ask for. This journey is overwhelming to do on your own. It can feel scary to face your fears without support. Generalizing these steps and tools into real life situations takes practice, persistence, and resiliency. Working with a coach will help you navigate the turbulent waters of caregiving and will keep hope alive for you and your loved one. It's natural to feel the tidal wave of emotions and a sense of helplessness. The idea that we have control over our lives disappears when we receive the news. Disease wasn't part of your life plan and dreams, and certainly, caring for your loved one's battle with the disease wasn't either.

As you're in this caregiving role, you're probably just beginning to figure out what questions you need to ask. Don't be surprised when the more answers you get, the more questions come to mind. Above all, don't expect that you'll know what to do right away. Your caregiving challenges will vary with the type and severity of the diagnosis. You'll have to wear multiple hats as you confront a host of situations. At times, you'll find yourself suddenly overwhelmed with conflicting urgent demands. This flurry of unexpected activities will be intensely frustrating.

Know that caregiving will test your physical health, stamina, patience, emotional stability, and commitment to your loved one many times over and in ways that are hard to imagine now. Some days you'll feel so overwhelmed, exhausted, and discouraged that you'd like nothing better than to throw in the towel, if only you had that option. This preview of the rollercoaster ride and the stresses you'll encounter along the way is not meant to discourage you on your caregiving journey. Rather, it's intended to encourage you to take a deep breath, activate your inner strength, buckle your seatbelt, and continue this journey with clearer expectations, an open mind, and an open heart.

It's possible to live your best life during this challenging phase. You can do it on your own, but it will be easier and sustainable when you hire a coach. I emphasize the importance of self-care and create the sacred space and environment for you to see yourself more clearly and flourish. I help you identify gaps between where you are and where you want to be with your wellness and loved one's journey. I help you identify and focus on what's important (this includes you and your wellbeing!), which accelerates your success. It helps to have someone in your corner who cares about you and makes sure you get the important things done.

In this process, you will be installing a new empowered belief system to replace the old, and you will be elevated to care for yourself too. You will experience deep transformations when you do the inner work. There is no better way to learn about dealing with a disease as a caregiver than by choosing a compassionate coach who shares their caregiver experience with you and provides you with a proven, reliable system of structure and support. It's not by chance you've picked up this book. I believe it's by divine appointment that you're reading this and we've met this way. Something bigger than ourselves guided us together. By sharing my experiences and wisdom with you, I trust that you will receive exactly what you need to help you and your loved one navigate this journey. My intention is for you to see your value and worth, to care for yourself as deeply as you care for your loved one, and live your best life because it's your birthright. *You're stronger than you think you are. You can do this!*

Chapter 13:

WOULD WORKING WITH A COACH BE HELPFUL?

You've gone through eight steps for preventing caregiver burnout. Hopefully, as you went through them, ideas came to mind, and you wrote them down. I see you. I hear you. I know what it feels like doing it all alone. This book will help you overcome your caregiving challenges when you do the work. This won't work if you simply close this book and store it on the shelf. My intention is for this information to be helpful and useful to you now, and in the future. You now have tools and *soul*utions to navigate and prevent caregiver burnout. The reality is you can probably do these steps on your own. The question is will you do them consistently?

Healing is about reflecting and looking at what has happened and saying that it will never defeat you. Here's an example of affirmations I've used when I have gone through tough times as a caregiver. "This will *never* defeat me. I am tuned into love. I will turn this into my source of wisdom and strength. I have the power to choose love, wisdom and peace. I choose sharing my wisdom to help others. I am on a mission to inspire others to live their best life during life's battles. I am changing the lives of caregivers, one caregiving heart at a time!"

What's Your Plan of Action?

Recall the definition of compassion fatigue that you read at the beginning. It's an extreme state of tension and preoccupation with the suffering of those being helped, to the degree that it can create a secondary traumatic stress for the helper. Often, caregivers don't stop to realize how stressful and unhappy they've become. Not you! You've read this book!

Here are some things you've learned:

1. *Soul*utions to caregiving problems.
2. That you're not alone and other caregivers, including myself, have had victory when they've asked for help.
3. The importance of partnering and effectively communicating with your loved one's health team.
4. How to create an effective schedule that ensures that you and your family have everything you need and nothing slips through the cracks.

5. Self-awareness of your mind, body, and spirit.
6. Tools and techniques to become compassion resilient.
7. Why self-care is critical to your success and your loved one's wellness journey.
8. Caregivers who bring refreshed, rejuvenated, and uplifted energy when caring for their loved ones bring hope and joy.

You have seen principles and strategies to prevent burnout. All you need now is a plan of action to put these principles into practice. Now is the time to put it all together and implement the plan of action. Schedule this plan in your calendar, and do it now!

What are the Benefits of Working with a Coach?

A compassionate, transformational coach helps to bridge the gap between what you know and what you do by:

- 💜 Working with you to help your loved one beat their disease.
- 💜 Providing accountability for the goals you set.
- 💜 Helping you communicate clearly with the doctors and prevent medical errors with your loved one's care.
- 💜 Providing extra support and resources when you need them.
- 💜 Helping you to stay strong and empowered so that you can give your loved one the support and care they need, no matter how hard it gets.

A compassionate coach will also help you:

- ♥ Get better, easier, faster, and sustainable results. Often, when we try to do things on our own, we fail and give up. You're not alone. You don't need to travel this road on your own.
- ♥ Become aware of your state of mind, body, and spirit.
- ♥ Learn tools and techniques to become compassion-resilient.
- ♥ Become super clear about why self-care is critical to your success and your loved one's wellness journey.
- ♥ Learn the power of gratitude, meditation, and journaling.
- ♥ Learn the power of acceptance and forgiveness.

Choosing to work with a coach is not a failure on your part. Instead, it's an expression of value for yourself by accepting support. Release the old thoughts of discouragement, and welcome new thoughts of joy and gratitude and, most of all, support. Invest in your best asset - *you*!

Seeking a coach is extremely beneficial and speeds up the process to breakthrough your limitations. They also help you move through the difficult moments that will arise during your journey. A coach will hold you accountable for your goals and help you get through the difficult and more anxious periods of your life, all while learning ways to navigate and help your loved one battle disease.

I tried to do all the work myself over the years. I read many self-help books, completed many courses and certifications, and dove deep into various healing modalities for over twenty years. What I've noticed is that I received the greatest, life-changing moments of success when I asked for support and hired a coach to help me on my journey, taking me to the next level.

When I invest in myself, exchange money for support, I'm accountable for my work. Proven systems of structure and support create the safe space for transformation to occur. We all face difficulties that are new to us and sometimes, repeat difficulties with the same results. In order to experience new results, a new level of awareness is required. A coach will help you become aware and help you achieve new outcomes.

Even coaches have coaches. I'm trained and know what to do, yet I still hire coaches as accountability partners to help me reach new levels, and bring in a new level of awareness. I am a trained professional who has gone through rigorous training and life experiences and who is passionate about improving the lives of my clients, to help them recognize that the Power within them is greater than any condition, situation, or circumstance. May You be empowered and live this journey with peace of mind.

ACKNOWLEDGMENTS

To fulfill my vision for this book, I needed access to caregivers, many of whom were in my immediate network circle and others who were referred by friends, family, and strangers. Some have become my clients, and I'm deeply grateful to share this journey with you.

I am grateful to my parents who provided me with the environment to learn ways to become a compassionate resilient caregiver. Thank you for believing in me. I also want to sincerely thank my brother, sisters, nieces, and nephews who've shared the caregiving experience. Without the collaboration and working together as a Petrolo team, this journey would have been more challenging.

To my first coaching client, I want to thank you for trusting me with your life. From our first conversation in the rainforest where you shared your experience as a caregiver for your sister, I knew we would have a life-long relationship. I am so proud of your commitment to yourself! It is an absolute gift and privilege to see your transformation and successes.

Thanks to my mentors, coaches, and thought leaders who continue to empower me with wisdom. There are too many people and too few pages here to thank everyone. I hesitate to name any if I cannot name all, but some people must be recognized for breathing new life into this project: Mary Morrissey and team at the Brave Thinking Institute, and Dr. Angela and team at The Author Incubator. As well, thank you to David Hancock and the Morgan James Publishing team for helping me bring this book to print.

I'll forever be grateful for my health care team of physicians, therapists, nurses, coaches, and healers. I want you to know how much I value your partnership, care, and insight on living my best life so that I vibrantly pursue my purpose. I appreciate you being there when I needed you.

To my friend Sue, who has been telling me for years that I needed to write a book; in fact, she has always encouraged me to write an encyclopedia set! (That's how far back this goes...) Thanks for your never-ending encouragement and support.

Special thanks to the caregivers who take care of my dog, plants, and home during my travels. You know who you are. ;) I am so grateful you're all in my life!

And finally, my deepest thanks to my sister Rose, my greatest partner in believing that all things are possible. Words cannot describe how grateful I am for your continuous support and love. I wouldn't be where I am without you.

In addition, I offer an apology. Although I have changed most of the details of the stories and many of the names for privacy, you may see yourself in this book. This book is not meant to hurt but to help and heal. It is written with love.

Once more, I offer a most profound gratitude to all of you who have contributed to writing this book and helping me pursue my mission to transform the lives of caregivers and their families, one caregiving heart at a time.

Each one of you is a magnificent light warrior!

CELEBRATION TIME!

Y ou have taken a great step towards living your best life with love, joy and grace while being a caregiver. Thank you for picking up this book and reading it!

How much you improve and how good you feel on this journey is directly related to the actions and attitude you have towards yourself. This means that the real work of living your best life depends on where you go from here. Simply reading this book isn't enough. You need to integrate the ideas and information into your life for things to change.

As a token of my appreciation for taking this great step for yourself, I am giving you two gifts. The first is a free video class. I have a companion video series that goes with this book. Send an email to info@josephinegracecoaching.com to sign up for it.

I'm also offering a free love and grace strategy session. If you're interested in embracing the challenge and *your* uniqueness with joy and grace, then schedule your appointment with me here: info@josephinegracecoaching.com.

May you find your life enriched in unpredictable ways by your caregiving experience.

Embrace. Love. Now.

ABOUT THE AUTHOR

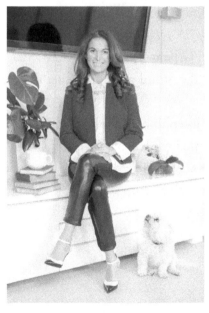

Josephine Grace is an international speaker and certified transformation life coach. She earned a dual degree, Honours in Bachelor of Arts and Social Science, and Bachelor of Education from the University of Toronto and continues to invest in advanced training and education. She has studied several healing modalities and personal development for the past 25 years and helps individuals, families, and professional caregivers create richer, more fulfilling lives. As a well-being advocate and caregiver for her parents, Josephine has real life experience with navigating health, grief, loss and acceptance which inspires others and help them live their best life. Her professional career includes business management, business development and educator. She is the best-selling author of *Help! My Loved One Has Cancer: 8 Steps to Prevent Caregiver Burnout.* Josephine lives in Southern Ontario, Canada and is the proud momma of her dog Lexi.

Connect with Josephine online at:
Website: www.thejoyfulcaregiver.com
Facebook: https://www.facebook.com/JosephineGraceAuthor
Instagram: @josephinegracecoach